HOW TO OVERCOME A BAD BACK

HOW TO OVERCOME
A BAD BACK

JAMES R. SHERMAN

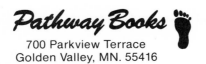
Pathway Books
700 Parkview Terrace
Golden Valley, MN. 55416

First Edition, February, 1980
Copyright© 1980 James R. Sherman
All Rights Reserved

Library of Congress Catalog Number
79-90870

International Standard Book Number:
0-935538-00-3

Pathway Books
700 Parkview Terrace
Golden Valley, MN 55416

To: Christopher, Eric, Lincoln, and Merlene

CONTENTS

ILLUSTRATIONS

FOREWORD

The symptom of low back pain is the most common complaint heard by physicians. In fact, there are few subjects in medicine that have stimulated as much experimental investigation and research to determine the cause and find a solution as the problem of low back pain. Medical literature on the subject is enormous. Much has been learned about the causes of low back pain from an anatomical, neurological, and biomechanical standpoint. But the medical profession has yet to solve the riddle of how to cure back pain. This is evident by the fact that so many patients treated medically or surgically for this symptom either fail to improve or are made worse by the treatment they receive. Until doctors find specific procedures that will guarantee a permanent cure in every case, the disabling symptom of back pain will continue to plague the human race.

As a surgeon who has spent a lifetime—over 40 years—operating on people with low back pain, I am honored to be asked to write a foreword to this book. I have read most of the medical literature on this subject and know of no writing that can compare with Dr. Sherman's work. The author, who is a nonmedical person, has presented to the sufferer of back pain a vast amount of practical information, crystalized from personal experience and study. He has described in depth how a disabling symptom can change a normal, strong, healthy, and self-sufficient and individual into a physical and psychological cripple. But just as thoroughly, he has set forth procedures for conquering those problems.

Dr. Sherman once suffered all of the agonies of a bad back. His autobiographical approach provides a vivid description of a disabling symptom, what it did to him, and what he did to overcome it. His philosophy is and has been: you don't have to live with your back problem—do something about it!

Dr. Sherman has described very clearly and in simple language the anatomy of the spine, how it works, how it is injured, and what parts become painful. He also describes methods of treatment that can bring temporary or permanent relief. The most valuable contribution he has made, however, is in analyzing and providing solutions to the personal problems of the back pain sufferer.

I predict that Dr. Sherman's book will become the "bible of back pain", to be used as a guide not only by disabled patients and their friends, associates, and employers, but also by the physicians who treat them.

Doctors who are too busy to really learn or understand the numerous ramifications of the disabilities their back patients must live with will find this book, as I did, an enlightening and valuable addition to their professional libraries.

RALPH B. CLOWARD, M.D.
Honolulu, Hawaii

PREFACE

For five years, my family and I fought to overcome back pain and its related problems. During that time, my wife and I each had the same three back operations—laminectomy, chemonucleolysis, and fusion. Together with our three sons, we had a total of 43 hospital admissions for back problems, knee surgery, hockey stitches, eye injuries, and other assorted calamities.

At one time, my wife and I were both in the hospital at the same time for treatment of our back problems. On another occasion, I took one son to the hospital for hockey stitches, while my wife was in a second hospital being fitted for a body cast and another son was in a third hospital having knee surgery.

We were treated by specialists in acupuncture, allergy, anesthesiology, chiropractic, eye surgery, gynecology, internal medicine, neurology, neurosurgery, orthopedic surgery, pediatrics, psychiatry, radiology, rheumatology, and urology.

When back problems were at their worst, I had to give up my job and was unemployed for six months. Social and sexual activities for my wife and I changed significantly. I became moderately addicted to drugs and alcohol, and I frequently contemplated suicide. I now join my sons in vigorous games of racquetball and golf, and I walk two miles or more each day.

During the five-year period, I looked everywhere I could for help. I found people who didn't care, but more surprising, I found people who didn't know what to do, including many doctors. I got the most help from people who had actually suffered back pain and disability—with one exception. My wife and I were able to overcome our bad backs with the help of a fantastic human being who has our nomination for the world's greatest neurosurgeon.

I learned a lot about my back during those years. I also learned how to overcome pain, disability, frustration, and anger. That's what prompted me to write this book.

It's addressed to each of the 7 million Americans who have bad backs and are searching for a complete and rapid recovery. I also wrote the book for several million other people who come in daily contact with bad-back sufferers and who are striving to understand the mysterious aspects of back problems.

This book provides guidelines for working through and conquering all of the major problems associated with bad backs. But it is meant to complement—not replace—competent professional care.

It takes hard work, faith, and perseverance to overcome back problems, and many bad-back sufferers find it difficult to do by themselves. If you are inclined to share your experiences, or if you have any questions about the material in this book, please don't hesitate to write to me. I would enjoy hearing from you.

JAMES R. SHERMAN, Ph.D.

ACKNOWLEDGEMENTS

Thanks to Barbara Baker and Helen Bowlin for their editorial reviews, and to Dorothy Seeber who typed the final manuscript.

Thanks also to our doctors, nurses, neighbors, and friends who did so much to help us get through some very traumatic times.

Finally, thanks to those special people in Hawaii who will forever be a part of me.

INTRODUCTION

Right now, 7 million Americans are being treated for back pain. Another 70 million people have already experienced some form of severe and prolonged back problem during their lifetime, and almost 2 million new cases are added each year. Your chances are 8 in 10 that you will suffer a crippling back problem at some point in your life.

Back pain, sometimes called lumbago, is second only to respiratory ailments as the most frequent reason people visit a doctor's office, and it leads headache as the most common form of chronic pain. A recent National Health Survey reported that Americans make 19 million visits each year to doctors' offices because of back problems. That's more visits than are made for the common cold.

TYPICAL BAD BACK VICTIMS

The typical person with a bad back is a male officeworker in his late thirties or early forties who is 20 to 30 pounds overweight, and who engages in little or no exercise. He is employed in a high pressure job that bothers him. He frequently experiences unusual amounts of stress and has difficulty in dealing with it.

Women usually experience back problems while still in their child-bearing years. Pregnancy and stress are two of the major causes of their back disorders.

Statistics have shown that people in higher economic levels are more likely to suffer bad backs than those who are less affluent. Geographically, people in the northern and western United States are twice as likely to have back problems as those living in the South.

Many people who suffer chronic back pain are either physically or psychologically dependent on one or more drugs. Unfortunately, this is due to the fact that many doctors find it easier to prescribe pain pills and/or tranquilizers than to try to identify and treat the underlying cause of back pain.

Even if you're not a typical bad-back victim, chances are your problems are due to one of several common causes.

CAUSES OF BACK PROBLEMS

Most bad backs are triggered by the last of a long series of events that have become part of a person's life style. Once a person has had a severe bad-back attack, a pattern of back problems has very likely been created that will last for several years. Some of the most common causes of bad backs are listed here.

1. *Congenital and Developmental Defects:* problems with bones and muscles that existed at birth, or developed gradually through the maturation process.

2. *Disc Disorders:* includes the "slipped", herniated, ruptured, and degenerated discs.

3. *Dislocations and Fractures:* includes displacement of vertebrae and broken backs, which are breaks in one or more vertebrae of the spinal column.

4. *Infections and Tumors:* includes osteoarthritis, which is wearing out of bone; rheumatoid arthritis, which is disease of the cartilage in a joint; and gouty arthritis, which results from excessive uric acid.

5. *Pregnancy:* includes difficulties that stem from weakening of stomach and back muscles and the compression of discs from swayback.

6. *Referred Pain:* the triggering of pain and muscle spasms in the area of the back as a result of painful disease or injury in another part of the body.

7. *Spondylolithesis:* the forward slipping of a spinal vertebrae upon the bone beneath it.

8. *Stress, Tension, and Fatique:* includes emotional problems that cause tightening and overextension of stomach and back muscles.

9. *Trauma:* includes injuries, blows to the back, compression of one or more discs, strains or sprains of muscles, and torn ligaments. Traumas may be sudden or chronic. The aggrevation of pain from sleeping on a bad mattress is an example of chronic trauma.

The most common causes of bad backs are acute injury, inadequate musculature, disc disorders, and psychological tension.

Controversy remains over which causes are most significant. A now-famous study of 5,000 patients with back pain was conducted in 1944 by New York University and Columbia-Presbyterian Hospital. It reported no evidence of bad discs, tumors, or other organic conditions in 80 percent of the patients. The cause of their pain was described as a combination of stress, tension, and inadequate or inflexible muscles and tendons. The study has not been replicated during the intervening 35 years, in spite of the fact that more sophisticated means of diagnosing back disorders have been developed.

A nationally-known specialist in rehabilitation and retraining of muscles believes about 95 percent of all back pain is the result of weak muscles. On the other hand, an equally renowned orthopedic surgeon, believes over 33 percent of all back pain is the result of degenerative disc disease. Other specialists have reported that emotions, stress, and tension have a significant impact on back pain.

The fact that bad backs constitute a major national health problem for a significant number of Americans, coupled with the fact that the causes are in dispute, points to the need for greater knowledge and understanding. The consequences of misdiagnosis or inappropriate treatment can be devastating for a person with back pain.

OUTLINE OF THIS BOOK

This book was written to help people understand bad backs, how they happen, and what can be done to overcome the pain and crippling effects they produce. It is intended to complement, not replace, competent professional care.

Part I describes the back and what can go wrong with bones, muscles, nerves, and emotions. It also describes the condition of pain, and the effects of aging.

Part II provides some helpful information on how to cope with life situations that are affected by back problems. Work, sex, marriage, doctors, drugs and alcohol, and daily functions are among the topics discussed.

Part III explains the ways in which bad backs are diagnosed and treated. Exercise, surgery, psychotherapy, relaxation, and other treatments are covered in detail.

Most of the statistical data and medical information found on these pages was extracted from one or more of the sources listed in the bibliography, which along with an index is found at the end of the book.

As complex as back problems are, it would take much more than is presented here to give you all the answers. But with this book, you are on the pathway to greater knowledge about your condition. Hopefully, it will be a productive journey.

PART I

YOUR BACK AND ITS PROBLEMS

1. WHAT YOU MUST KNOW ABOUT YOUR BACK

Overcoming bad-back problems is not an easy task. So much depends on what you can and are willing to do for yourself. That's why you need to know and understand everything you can about how your back is put together. You must also know about the psychological factors that are associated with back problems. If you don't know these things, your recovery will take much longer and be more difficult.

Fear of the unknown is one of life's most insidious adversaries. If you are suffering pain you don't clearly understand, then you probably are frightened by the prospect of permanent disability, continued mental anguish, fantasized surgeries, or other calamities. But the more you learn about your back, the less you will have to fear.

Knowledge about the structure and function of your mind and body will allow you to converse intelligently with those you depend on for treatment. If you don't know what's going on, you may be catapulted into accepting treatments you won't be able to understand, and your anxiety over the unknown may make your problems worse. Conversely, your fear and lack of knowledge might cause you to refuse treatments that could ensure a rapid recovery.

You need to know about the bones in your back, because they provide the framewok for your body. You need to understand about discs, because they may possibly be at the root of your back problems. You need to identify the location and function of the muscles in your back, because that's the key to your recovery. You need to know about ligaments, because they tie the parts of your back together. You need to know how your nervous system transmits sensations of pain, and how it can suffer damage from protruding discs. You need to know about the nature of pain so you can cope with it and not let it take over your life. You need to know how your mind reacts to back problems so you can control disruptive thoughts. Finally, you need to know about the crises of life that can bring on or accentuate back problems.

The material included in part Part I provides the foundation for a complete understanding of our back and its problems. It covers most of what you need to know to start on your road to recovery. A separate chapter is devoted to each of the major parts of your back, beginning with the spinal column.

2. THE SPINAL COLUMN

The spinal column—also called the vertebral column, spine, or backbone—is the most important part of your back. In addition to supporting your head and ribs, your spinal column provides a conduit for your your nervous sysem. But even though it is the most central structural member of your body, it must be held upright by muscles and ligaments.

This chapter describes the nature and arrangement of the spinal column and its supporting elements. It explains how bones grow and repair themselves, and it presents three of the many bone-related problems that can affect your back.

ARCHITECTURE OF THE SPINE

Your spinal column consists of 33 bones called vertebrae that are stacked one above the other between your hip and your head. The 33 vertebrae, of which 24 are movable, are commonly classified into five groups. Each vertebra within a group is shaped a little differently from the rest to serve specific purposes.

Starting at the top in the region of your neck are the seven cervical vertebrae. They are smaller than the others, and their chief purpose is to help you move your head.

The 12 thoracic vertebrae are located right below the cervical vertebrae. They are the ones to which your ribs are attached. Together with the ribs, they enclose and protect your lungs and heart.

Next in line are the five lumbar vertebrae—the workhorses of the spine. They are the biggest vertebrae because they handle most of the stress placed on your back. They are also involved in most back problems. Their size enables them to serve as the fulcrum of the body; a hinge for lifting objects of all sizes.

The five sacral vertebrae are found right below the lumbar vertebrae. They are fused together into one bone called the sacrum. They rest on the pelvis where they form a bridge between your spine and your legs.

At the very bottom of the spinal column are the four vertebrae of the coccyx, which are also fused together into one bone called the tailbone. This bone is, in turn, fused to the sacrum above it. The coccyx is called the tailbone because it probably is all that remains of the tail humans may have possessed in their early stages of evolution.

Doctors use a combination of letters and numbers to describe positions on the spinal column. L4-L5 indicates the space between your fourth and fifth lumbar vertebrae. L5-S1 indicates the space between your fifth lumbar and first sacral vertebrae. These two regions are where most back problems occur, so these designations are used quite often. All of your vertebrae are numbered in groups from the top down as shown in figure 1.

Your vertebrae are securely bound together, and to other bones, by ligaments. They are also attached to muscles by tendons. The fact that your vertebrae are not locked together allows for twisting, bending, and other body movements.

Instead of being stacked straight up and down, your vertebrae form characteristic curves. When you were a baby, your spine had a round, backward curve from the pelvis to the skull. As you grew and began to stand upright, your spine developed subcurves. As an adult, your spine now curves forward in the neck region, backward in the chest area, and forward again in the lower back. By tilting your pelvis forward the curves are accentuated, resulting in an unsatisfactory condition called swayback or lordosis as shown in figure 2. Backward tilting of your pelvis tends to straighten out the curves of your spine.

Your stomach and back muscles keep the middle of your spine over your body's center of gravity. Since movement of the spine is greatest in the lower back, this region is the one that suffers the greatest number of problems.

Each vertebra has a hole in the middle like a doughnut. The column

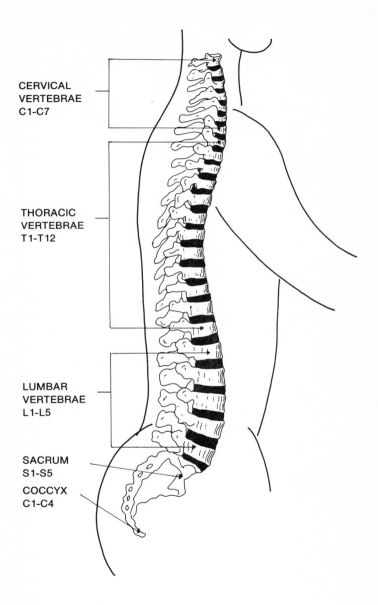

CERVICAL
VERTEBRAE
C1-C7

THORACIC
VERTEBRAE
T1-T12

LUMBAR
VERTEBRAE
L1-L5

SACRUM
S1-S5

COCCYX
C1-C4

FIGURE 1. THE SPINAL COLUMN

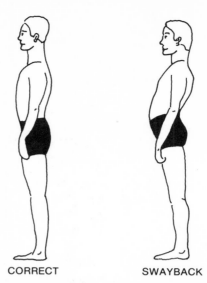

CORRECT   SWAYBACK

FIGURE 2. CORRECT AND SWAYBACK POSTURE

of holes that is formed through the 33 vetebrae is called the spinal canal. Passing down through this canal from the brain is your spinal cord, consisting of nerve cells that send and recieve impulses from all parts of your body.

There are 31 pairs of nerves branching out from your spinal cord through the space between each pair of vertebrae. One set of nerves goes to the left side of your body, and the other set goes to the right side. The nerves that run down your legs, for example, join the spinal cord between two vertebrae in the lumbar region. That explains why pain is often felt in the legs and feet when the back goes bad.

Separating the bony vertebrae are cushions of elastic cartilage called discs (also spelled disks). The discs absorb shocks and permit your vertebrae to bend and twist without grating on each other. If your discs were not there to serve as cushions, each vertebra would grind against the one above and below as your body moved. The nerves, which would be caught in the middle, would send out excruciating pain.

There are four, short, finger-like extensions pointing upward and downward on either side of your vertebrae, as shown in figures 3 and 4. At the end of each extension is a smooth, oval surface called the

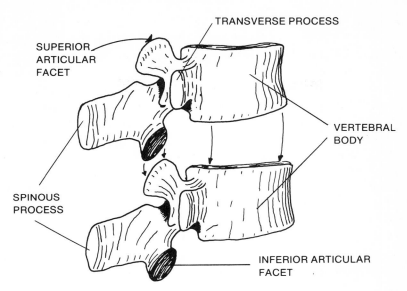

FIGURE 3. VERTEBRAE-SIDE VIEW

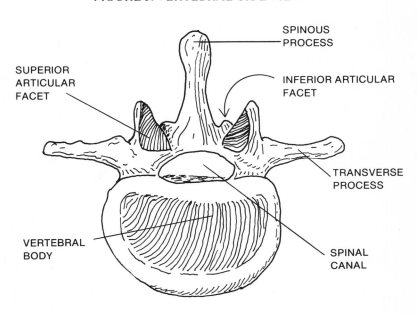

FIGURE 4. TOP VIEW OF LUMBAR VERTEBRA

articular facet. This surface joins with a similar bone on the vertebrae above and below—two against the upper and two against the lower. The joints themselves are encased in ligaments and tissue much like other bone joints in your body. When your back moves, these bony surfaces rub against and support each other. Normally, most of your weight is distributed on the main body of the vertebra and on the intervertebral discs. The articular facets usually act only as stabilizers.

Extending backward from the main body of your vertebrae is an elongated piece of bone called the spinous process. Together, the spinous processes of all the vertebrae make up the bony ridge you can feel when you rub your hand up and down your back.

As you can see, your back is a very complex part of your body. You can develop serious problems if any of the interrelated components are impaired in some way. Your spinal column is particularly vulnerable because it is central to so many functions.

BONE CHEMISTRY

The process by which bones grow and repair themselves is very important for someone with a bad back, especially in cases where fusion is contemplated. Vertebrae are frequently fused together to repair broken backs or replace herniated discs. As you might expect, the bones in your spinal column are a lot like other bones in your body. Disregarding water, they consist of two-thirds mineral and one-third organic matter.

Nearly all bone surfaces are covered by a tough membrane called the periosteum. Bone cells receive nourishment from blood vessels that weave through the periosteum and reach the spongy interior, either directly or through an intricate network of tiny canals. Nerve fibres follow similar routes.

Bone grows and repairs itself in fascinating ways. When a bone is broken, lacerated tissues pour out a sticky, oozy substance that stiffens into a bulgy deposit. Little by little, bone-making cells and fractured bone ends penetrate the substance and replace it with spongy bone to hold the injured parts more firmly in place. Bone-dissolving cells gradually remove the spongy bone and replace it with hard bone. This process also occurs when bones are fused together, either by surgery or by intense compression.

Knowledge of bone chemistry is also important for dealing with such back disorders as spondylolithesis, scoliosis, and spondylitis.

SPONDYLOLITHESIS

Sometimes, a lumbar vertebra will slip forward and down on to the vertebra below it. Intense pain will result when the bones rub together and irritate adjoining nerves. This painful condition is called spondylolithesis. It usually results from a congenital or early developmental defect, and it occurs in 5 to 7 percent of the population. It can also exist without pain, and is sometimes discovered by accident. The defect is most common with the L5 vertebra, but does occur at L4 as well. Pain, usually felt in the low back, often radiates into both buttocks and the upper thighs.

The symptoms of spondylolithesis closely resemble those of disc disorders. Many times, conservative treatment for a bad disc masks the underlying spondylolithesis. If the downward slip of the vertebrae is extensive, the spine may have to be fused. But without pain and other symptoms, many teenagers and young adults lead perfectly normal lives, despite their spondylolithesis.

SCOLIOSIS

Scoliosis is the name given to the unnatural, and sometimes sideways, curvature of the spine. If the problem occurs because of postural defects, correction can usually be done quite easily. It is much more difficult, however, to straighten scoliosis that is due to structural abnormalities. There are several types of scoliosis, of which three are most common.

1. *Idiopathic Scoliosis.* This condition begins in childhood and gets progressively worse until growth ceases.

2. *Structural Scoliosis.* This type of scoliosis can be due to abnormally shaped vertebrae, or it can come from other causes, such as muscular weakness resulting from polio.

3. *Sciatic Scoliosis.* This problem lasts only as long as some

primary condition of the spine produces muscle spasms to protect an area of the back that hurts. By far, the most common cause of sciatic scoliosis is the herniation or rupture of an intervertebral disc. Abnormal posture occurs involuntarily as the body attempts to minimize pain and discomfort. People with sciatic scoliosis tend to favor the painful areas and end up leaning to one side. Once the underlying disc problem is resolved, normal posture is restored.

SPONDYLITIS

Spondylitis is a progressive disease caused by a bacterial infection. It fuses the small joints of the spine and calcifies the long spinal ligaments. When seen on X-ray, spondylitis makes the spine appear as though it was composed of bamboo.

Spondylitis may be arrested at any stage with medications. In a few patients it may progress slowly until the entire spine from head to pelvis is immobilized. At that point, breathing is very difficult since inhibited rib movement prevents the chest from expanding.

Treatment of spondylitis involves the use of medications such as aspirin and a program of posture-correcting exercises. If the bones become deteriorated and lose their support functions, fusion will have to be done.

Spondylolithesis, scoliosis, and spondylitis are back disorders that involve the vertebrae. More commonly, back pain and disability result from deterioration of the intervertebral discs as explained in the next chapter.

3. DISCS

Discs are cartilaginous cushions that are located between the bony vertebrae in your spinal column. Although basically quite simple in structure and function, discs can be the source of very serious problems when they deteriorate.

This chapter describes the structure of discs, as well as the nature and cause of disc problems.

DISC ANATOMY

Intervertebral discs are about 1¾ inches across at the widest point, and between ¼- and ⅜-inches thick. The outside of a disc looks somewhat like a radial tire. It consists of very tough cartilaginous tissue, but it is elastic enough to conform to the pressures placed on it. When you move from side-to-side or from front-to-back you tend to squash the discs. When you straighten up, the discs rebound to their normal shape.

Figure 5 shows the placement of a disc between two vertebrae.

Discs have an outer fibrous covering called the *annulus fibrosis*. The covering is about ⅛-inch thick, and completely encases the soft, pulpy core of the disc called the *nucleus pulposes*. The core has the consistency of Jello-O pudding, its liquid content gives it the capability to absorb shocks.

Like other ligaments, the annulus fibrosis is attached firmly to the vertebrae above and below it as shown in figure 6. As the ligament stretches, it allows movement of your spine, but it will only stretch so far. When you bend forward, backward, or side-to-side, the ligament acts as a restraint. Inside, your discs act as water-filled

18

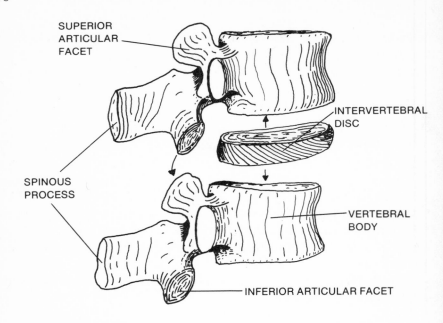

SUPERIOR
ARTICULAR
FACET

INTERVERTEBRAL
DISC

SPINOUS
PROCESS

VERTEBRAL
BODY

INFERIOR ARTICULAR FACET

FIGURE 5. POSITION OF DISC BETWEEN VERTEBRAE

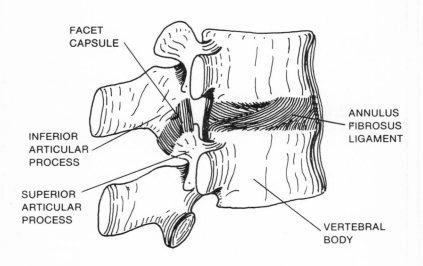

FACET
CAPSULE

ANNULUS
FIBROSUS
LIGAMENT

INFERIOR
ARTICULAR
PROCESS

SUPERIOR
ARTICULAR
PROCESS

VERTEBRAL
BODY

FIGURE 6. TWO VERTEBRAE JOINED
BY LIGMENTS

balloons. When you bend forward, the inside pulp is compressed to the back. When you bend backwards, the pulpy core is compressed forward. The core can bulge in almost any direction, but it cannot get outside the ligament. Unless, of course, the ligament has a crack in it, which it sometimes does.

DISC DISORDERS

As you get older, the annulus fibrosis can weaken and develop cracks or tears. Excessive stress on a disc can compress the inside pulp against the weakened outer covering so that a bulge occurs. This is called a herniated disc, and it is much like the bulge of an inner tube through a tire casing.

The annulus fibrosis is thinner and weaker at the back of a disc, which is closer to your spinal canal and spinal nerves. Bulging of a disc usually occurs at this already weakened area, so chances are it will squeeze one of your nerves against a neighboring bone as shown in figure 7. That's when you start developing severe back pain.

Sometimes a bulge breaks completely through the outer covering and goes out into the spinal canal where the main spinal nerves are found. This is called a ruptured or an extruded disc. It is also called a slipped disc, although nothing has actually slipped.

The protruding bulge of a ruptured disc will generally press against one of the nerves coming off your spinal cord. As the nerve gets squeezed, you start feeling pain, numbness, feelings of pins and needles penetrating your skin, burning, or other sensations. These feelings will occur in your buttocks, low back, down one or both of your legs, into your ankles, and even into the balls of your feet. For some people, the pain feels as though a red-hot rod has been driven up through the bottom of one foot, all the way into the hip. It may also feel as though your ankles have been wrapped in barbed wire. The pain that travels down the sciatic nerve in your legs is known as sciatica, sciatic pain, or sciatic neuritis. If herniation occurs between cervical vertebrae in the neck region, the pain and numbness will be felt in your arms and hands.

If the annulus fibrosis ruptures completely, the herniated nucleus may protrude far enough, and create sufficient nerve pressure to cause weakness, loss of reflexes, or complete loss of sensation in

20

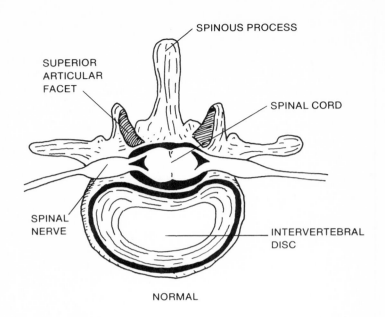

SPINOUS PROCESS

SUPERIOR
ARTICULAR
FACET

SPINAL CORD

SPINAL
NERVE

INTERVERTEBRAL
DISC

NORMAL

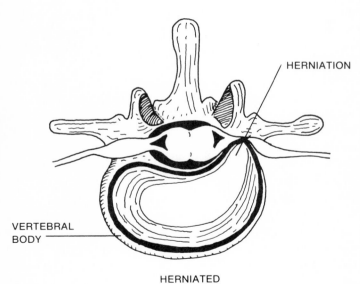

HERNIATION

VERTEBRAL
BODY

HERNIATED

FIGURE 7. NORMAL AND HERNIATED DISC

certain areas of your feet and legs. Crippling of your leg muscles will be accompanied by excruciating pain.

Not all back pain or sciatica is caused by a ruptured disc. Spinal cord tumors, vertebral joint deformities or dislocations, severe spinal arthritis, and other conditions can also give rise to back pain that radiates down the legs. But when a bulging disc is the culprit, the results are fairly predictable.

DYNAMICS OF BAD DISCS

The bulging of a disc and the rupture of the annulus fibrosis may happen suddenly from a specific trauma or stress, or through a slow process of degeneration. A disc may be so degenerated that a simple movement like bending over to tie your shoes can cause the disc to bulge into the spinal canal.

After people reach 20 years of age, it is normal for their discs to begin gradual degeneration. Early degeneration of discs does not cause bad-back symptoms unless some strain is added. The strain can be slight but prolonged, like sitting through a long automobile trip without stopping for rest or to stretch tired muscles. Even then, a doctor's examination may reveal only occasional pain and discomfort, along with mild tenderness in the back. X-rays might show nothing abnormal.

Disc disorders can also come from hard work in the yard, excessive lifting, or bending the wrong way; all of which add stress to your discs. If your discs are already in a stage of degeneration, a sudden and excessive stress can cause one or more to rupture.

Degenerative disc disease differs from an acute disc herniation in that it affects people in an older age range, and more often causes back pain rather than leg pain.

Disc problems occur because of degeneration of either the inner pulpy core, or the outer covering. When the inner core degenerates, through age or repeated and excessive stress, it loses its jelly-like consistency. It either becomes watery, which facilitates bulging; or it dries out, which makes it fibrous and less able to rebound after compression.

Studies have revealed that 20 percent of the people from 14 to 34 years of age have degenerated discs. Almost 75 percent of the people from 35 to 59 years of age, and 95 percent of the people over 60 years of age have abnormal discs. Discs can be abnormal without causing problems, unless they herniate into the spinal canal.

Of the people who do end up with herniated discs, about 15 percent are under 30 years of age, 67 percent are in their forties and fifties, and another 18 percent are over 50 years old. The ratio of males to females with disc problems is almost 79 to 21 percent.

The dynamics of bulging discs are not the same for all people. If the spinal canal is large, there may be plenty of room for both the nerves and the bulging disc. If the canal is small, even a slight bulge can cause extreme pain. Sometimes a bulge slips back within the outer covering before any serious damage is done. If the stress that caused the bulge is removed, the bulge may never occur again. Sometimes a bulge gets squeezed at the point where it comes through the outer covering. The bulge may separate, like a glob of toothpaste, and fall harmlessly into the spinal canal where it will disappear into the body structure. If a bulge stays out and continues to press against a spinal nerve, it must be removed surgically, or else it will kill the nerve.

About 9 out of 10 herniated or ruptured discs occur within the two lowest disc spaces in the spine. This would be between the fourth and fifth lumbar vertebrae, and between the fifth lumbar and the first sacral vertebrae. Using doctors' coding, the problems would be located at the L4-L5 and the L5-S1 levels. The problems occur here, because this is the area of the back that experiences the most stress. Doctors have reported that 80 percent of all disc problems occur at the L5-S1 level, 19 percent occur at the L4-L5 level, and the remaining 1 percent occur elsewhere in the spine.

In about 1 out of 10 cases, a double herniation occurs at two levels. This means that two discs are herniating at the same time. About 73 percent of the double herniations occur at the L4-L5 and L5-S1 levels. Almost all the rest occur at the L4-L5 and L3-L4 levels.

Sometimes, two bulges occur in the same disc. This probably would affect the nerves in both legs, but it would not be considered a double herniation.

About 30 percent of the herniated disc problems occur again if conservative treatment is followed and surgery is not performed. About 10 to 20 percent of the people who have a herniated disc need surgery. If surgery is not performed when it is indicated, a patient will suffer progressive nerve damage and possible paralysis in the legs.

Evidence proves that deteriorated discs cause painful and serious back problems. Many experts maintain, however, that condition of the muscles has a far greater impact on back pain and disability. The role that muscles play in back problems is discussed in the next chapter.

4. MUSCLES

The importance of muscles cannot be overemphasized, since more back problems occur because of poor muscle condition than any other cause. Conversely, improvement of muscle condition is probably the most effective and least expensive way of overcoming a bad back.

This chapter describes the nature and function of your back muscles and the need for maintaining proper muscle tone. Muscle damage and muscle spasms are also discussed.

MUSCLE FRAMEWORK

The importance of muscle condition is highlighted by the fact that about 150 muscles are attached to your spinal column. Some of them run parallel to the spine and hold your body erect. Others allow your body to rotate as they hold up your spine. Still others keep your stomach muscles from sagging, which reduces stress on your back.

Four major muscle groups work together to support your back. When one group is weakened, others have to carry the additional stress. If you can become knowledgeable about the structure and role of these muscle groups, you will have a distinct advantage in overcoming your bad back by strengthening those that are causing localized problems.

Abdominal Muscles. These muscles support your abdominal wall. They extend from the rib cage to the sides and front of your pelvis and are attached to these bony structures by tendons.

The abdominal muscles support the contents of your abdominal cavity, including your liver, gall bladder, stomach, small and large intestines, pancreas, spleen, bladder, kidneys, and sex organs. Not only are the abdominal muscles essential in providing support for your back, but as you can see, they are also called upon to protect some very important parts of your body.

Extensor Muscles. These muscles lie along, and are attached to your spine. They are also attached to your pelvis, ribs, and head. They are used in arching your back, in holding your spine still and erect, and in pulling weighted objects.

Lateral Muscles. These muscles run along the side of the spine and help control bending to one side. The muscles in this group are some of the largest in your body. They affect not only your back, but your hips as well.

Hip Muscles. Four subgroups of hip muscles are important to the function of your spine and hips. The muscles of one subgroup lie along the front of your hips and are used to bring your thighs upward when you try to step over an object. A second subgroup lies along the side of the hip from the top of your pelvis to your thigh bone. They provide stability for the hip and help you do such things as stand on one foot.

Your groin muscles make up a third subgroup that is used to pull your legs together at the knee and thigh. The fourth subgroup includes the massive muscles in your buttocks. They are the main muscles used in running, walking, climbing stairs, and maintaining good posture. The hamstring muscles that run down the back of your thigh from the pelvis are part of this fourth subgroup.

It's not enough just to know the location and function of the major muscle groups. It's also important to make sure your muscles can respond when called upon for support of your back.

MAINTAINING MUSCLE TONE

Your muscles will remain in good condition only if they are used. If you allow your muscles to become weak, they will be more susceptible to injury, and they will cause other parts of your body to be more vulnerable to a variety of problems.

It's important for you to know which muscles are involved in sitting, standing, lifting, walking, and other activities. You can then call on your stronger muscles to ease the burden of weak or sore and tender muscles. In exercising, you should pay special attention to those muscle groups that can do the most to help you overcome your bad back.

Kinesiologists (scientists who study the movement of parts of the body) have calculated the amount of energy expended by muscles when the body goes through normal movements. For example, if a man of average height, weighing 180 pounds, leans forward 60 degrees at the waist, the muscles in and around the back must exert a force of 450 pounds per square inch to keep him from falling on his face. If that same man were holding a weight of 50 pounds in his outstretched arms, his back muscles would have to exert a force of 750 pounds to keep him standing upright. If the man were to lift the 50 pound weight while holding it out from his body, a force of 850 pounds per square inch would be exerted on the fifth lumbar vertebra.

Weakness of the abdominal muscles is one of the most common causes of back problems. In ordinary movements, strong abdominal muscles keep the stomach from sagging forward and imposing dangerous stress on the lumbar region of the spine. In some cases, strengthening of the abdominal muscles may be all that's necessary to eliminate backaches.

When the abdominal muscles are not exercised, their neglect is very obvious. The once-taunt stretch of muscles across the stomach tends to sag, causing an unsightly potbelly. As the stomach expands, the intestines begin to uncoil and fill up the additional space. If the internal organs are not firmly packed into the stomach cavity, they become less efficient. Gas forms, causing the stomach to expand even further. The only way the abdominal cage can expand is forward, so the potbelly gets larger.

It's important to remember that your abdominal muscles help to support your spine. As the abdominals weaken, their supportive functions are assumed by other muscles in your sides and back. If other muscles have been as neglected as the abdominals, your spine will weaken from lack of support, pressure will be placed on potentially weakened discs, and herniation and back pain will occur.

Exercise alone will not correct the problems of weakened abdominal muscles and an unsightly potbelly, nor will exercise reduce the excess fat that is characteristically present. Only a rigorous combination of exercise and diet will reduce the potbelly and add necessary strength to the abdominal muscles.

MUSCLE DAMAGE

Back pain is generally caused either by acute injury or by degeneration of the joints, ligaments, muscles, or intervertebral discs. The most common injuries involve sprains and strains of muscles in and around the back.

Acute Muscle Sprain. A sudden bending of the spine from a fall or a sudden lifting motion can cause acute back sprain. Ligaments or membranes enclosing the joints are torn, muscle tissues become engorged with fluid, and blood flows from torn vessels. The fluids and inflamed tissues press against nerves, causing intense pain and protective muscle spasms. Sprains take a long time to heal because torn muscles are involved. The torn tissues will either heal after a long period of rest, in which case fibrous scar tissue will form, or they will have to be mended surgically. In most cases, however, new muscle cells are added to replace damaged ones.

A sprain in the ligaments of a disc will leave scar tissue that may press against the spinal nerves. This condition can be confused with a herniated disc, because the symptoms are much the same. Like a herniated disc, the scar tissue may have to be removed surgically to eliminate pain.

Acute Muscle Strain. When muscles, tendons, or ligaments are stretched beyond their normal limits, the back will suffer an acute strain. In a severe strain, inflamed tissues will become congested with fluids that will exert pressure on nerves and cause extreme pain. Tendons, which attach muscles to bones, can also be strained. Again, fluid buildup can cause intense pain in the back and legs. The tissues will mend after a period of rest and proper care while excess fluids are absorbed by the body.

Chronic Back Strain. Sometimes back strain doesn't come on suddenly as in an injury or accident. Instead, the structures in the back are subjected to prolonged stress and tension greater than they can endure. Symptoms come on gradually and get progressively worse over time. The condition is made even worse by fatigue.

The causes of chronic back strain make it difficult to treat. It can be brought on by living habits, such as sleeping the wrong way on a soft mattress. It can also be brought on by conditions of employment, such as driving heavy trucks, operating heavy equipment, or sitting at a desk for long periods. Constant stress and muscle tension can also bring on chronic back strain. If the cause cannot readily be removed, prognosis is very poor. A significant change in lifestyle is, in most cases, the only really effective cure, although improvement may be obtained through rest and physiotherapy.

Sprains and strains of muscles require fairly long recovery periods. If you become impatient and try to speed the recovery process, you will probably cause additional damage. Fortunately, muscle spasms serve as your body's alarm system to get you to stop punishing weak or damaged muscles.

MUSCLE SPASMS

Almost everyone has experienced a muscle spasm of some kind at one time or another. If you suffered a muscle spasm in your back, it probably was very severe and may have felt like someone stuck a knife or slammed an axe into your back muscles. Movement may have been impossible because of the intense pain.

Sometimes, spasms occur when bending over, making it impossible to straighten up. Inability to move may cause a person to feel that something is stuck, or that two bones are locked together. When describing the condition, people often refer to a "catch" in the back. In most cases, a muscle spasm is the culprit, and nothing is caught or stuck.

A muscle spasm is an involuntary, sustained contraction of a muscle that may occur when a nerve root becomes irritated. The resulting pain triggers muscles into tight contraction to protect the nerve and shield it against further irritation. This is the body's protective way of stopping people from continuing to abuse a bad condition. If excess stress is being placed on a weakened disc, for example, and if the disc is herniating against a spinal nerve, contraction of back muscles into spasm can prevent movement and stop the person from continuing the stressful activity.

Muscle spasms are caused by a lack of nutrition and a disruption of muscle cell metabolism. Normally, blood carries oxygen and other nutrients to the muscle cells through arteries. The blood leaves the muscle cells through veins, carrying with it metabolic waste products. The exchange takes place in thin-walled vessels called capillaries.

When muscles contact, the capillaries are squeezed shut. Ordinarily, the contractions are over quickly and the exchange of bodily materials is immediate. But when a muscle is in spasm, the contractions are prolonged, and the exchange cannot take place. The waste products, containing lactic acid, build up in the muscle cells and cause extreme pain. Pain also comes from starvation of the muscles, which are working very hard when in contraction. When the spasm is broken, blood flow returns to normal, the muscle cells are nourished, and wastes are removed.

If a muscle is injured or strained, surrounding muscles will form a splint around the nerves to protect them from further irritation. A "charley horse" is a muscle spasm that arises from excessive stress placed on muscles in an arm or a leg.

Sometimes the body tends to be overprotective and too many spasms occur. Continued contraction of muscles without relief causes extreme pain that radiates to other nerves, sending other muscles into protective spasm. The situation is common to bad-back attacks and is characterized by vicious pain cycles, multiple contractions, and repeated muscle spasms.

Muscle spasms can be brought on by sudden movement that irritates a ligament, muscle, or tendon in the back and results in an acute strain or sprain. Muscle spasms can also come from chronic back strain as "the final straw that broke the camel's back".

A person with a bad back can easily be identified. Widespread pain causes unaffected muscles to contract in order to help muscles that are hurting. This condition, called sciatic scoliosis, causes a person to list to one side while walking in order to accommodate the contracting muscles. The characteristic walk will stay with a person until the muscles heal.

Several steps can be taken to stop a muscle spasm. The first is to stop doing whatever caused the initial pain. You should lie down or find a suitably comfortable position to try to remove the precipitating stress. Normally, rest will enable the whole process to reverse itself. Your muscles will relax, the pain of muscle contraction will diminish, nerves will be less irritated, and finally, only residual pain will be felt.

Unfortunately, stopping a painful muscle spasm usually takes more time than many people are willing to give. They will either panic or get mad. Then they may scurry about trying to find someone or something that can help to ease their pain. Many times, however, the muscle spasm becomes so severe they are literally placed in a body cast by the contracting muscles. But immobilization is nature's way of preventing continued movement and avoiding irritation of additional muscles and nerves. If relief seems unlikely following rest, a doctor must be called to provide muscle-relaxing medication that will break the spasm.

Sometimes, pain and muscle spasm may be relieved as suddenly as they are brought on if the body is manipulated, either deliberately or accidently. Chiropractic adjustments and surgical reductions are deliberate manipulations, as is traction and immobilization of the spine. Deliberate manipulation must be done with extreme care to avoid damage to the spinal cord or the peripheral nerves. It should never be done without being preceded by a thorough diagnosis that is done by a qualified practitioner.

Accidental manipulation may cause disc fragments or herniated discs to suddenly shift, stopping irritation of a nerve. In other cases, a nerve can be irritated when the outer surfaces of a disc are pinched between two vertebrae. When the pinching stops from accidental manipulation, so does the irritation, spasm, and pain.

Heat and rest may help keep muscles relaxed so they don't go into spasm. Heat helps dilate blood vessels, allowing them to provide a richer supply of blood, oxygen, and food to the muscle tissues and remove pain-causing lactic acid waste. Heat liniments and ointments are generally not very effective because they can't reach deep enough beneath the skin surface to warm the affected muscles.

Warm showers and whirlpool baths (hydrotherapy) also help soothe tight and troubled muscles. Warm baths may be difficult, however, because of the stress of sitting, or of getting in and out of a bathtub.

Although muscle spasms can be triggered by injury or excessive stress, they can also be induced or compounded by emotional tension. The spasm and pain are continued because tension prevents the muscles from relaxing. Exercise can relieve emotional tension and help soothe muscles through relaxation and contraction.

Herniated discs produce characteristic muscle spasms that can only be broken through rest and medication. The dynamics of muscle spasms that accompany disc herniation are quite common and follow this general pattern.

1. Excessive pressure is exerted on a disc that is already weakened or unable to withstand the degree of stress that is involved.

2. The nucleus pulposes bulges through the annulus fibrosis and pinches spinal nerves or nerves in the outer disc layers.

3. The irritated nerve sends messages to the adjacent muscle giving it a jolt of pain.

4. The muscle contracts to protect the affected nerve.

5. Pain impulses from the contracted muscle may return to the irritated nerve which then sends out additional pain impulses.

6. The cycle of jolting pain from the nerves to contracting muscles and back to nerves, is so intense it becomes completely immobilizing. The sufferer cannot move and will collapse or lie down in extreme pain.

Muscles serve a great many of your body's needs. They do your work for you and protect you from danger. When you've abused your body and your actions threaten it with further injury, your muscles will go into spasm, forcing you to stop. Your muscles are clearly the most significant participant in your back problems.

5. LIGAMENTS

Ligaments don't sound as important as the other parts of your back, but if they're damaged through injury or deterioration, they can be the precipitating factor for many back problems. They are, as a matter of fact, the gateway through which herniated discs emerge.

Ligaments are thick, dense, and very tough strands of tissue that hold your skeleton together and keep your bones in place by attaching one bone to another. Ligaments are often confused with tendons, which are similar in structure and function, but which attach muscles to bones.

This chapter identifies the most important ligaments in your back, and describes what can happen when ligaments are damaged.

BACK LIGAMENTS

Back problems are generally associated with five major groups of ligaments, each of which is described below.

Interspinous Ligaments. These ligaments connect the spinous processes; the posterior extensions of vertebrae located in the middle of your spine that can be felt when you rub your hand along your back from top to bottom. The interspinous ligaments relax when you bend backwards and tighten up when you bend forward. They can be torn or ruptured if the body is thrown forward suddenly, as in a car accident.

Intertransverse Ligaments. These ligaments run along the sides of the vertebrae and keep you from bending too far to one side. They are very strong in the lumbar region of the back.

Ligamentum Flavum. These ligaments connect the rear parts of the vertebrae and help to cover and protect the spinal canal and the delicate nerve roots within.

Annulus Fibrosus. (See Discs) These ligaments connect each vertebra to the one above and below it. They form the outer layers of the intervertebral discs, prevent excessive movement of the vertebrae, and keep the discs in place. These ligaments are composed of several strong fibers that are interlaced at angles to each other and run in circular fashion like the strands of a radial-ply automobile tire. When they crack or tear because of age or injury, they leave a person vulnerable to a herniated or ruptured disc. It is through these ligaments that a ruptured disc will emerge into the spinal canal.

Anterior and Posterior Longitudinal Ligaments. These two ligaments extend from the top of your spine in your neck to the sacrum in your pelvis. One ligament covers the front of the vertebrae, and the other covers the back. Together, they constitute the outer wrap of the spine. As they cross between two vertebrae, they combine with and help to strengthen the annulus fibrosus.

Facet Capsule. Vertebrae are connected together by the disc in front and the articular facets behind. These facets are boney plates, which slide on each other when the spine moves forward and backward. They are tightly connected by a strong envelope of ligaments called the facet capsule, which stretches with spinal movements. Like other ligaments, the capsule may tear if you stretch too far.

Although there is little you can do to take care of your ligaments, it's important to know and understand their role in back problems, especially if they sustain serious damage.

LIGAMENT DAMAGE

If ligaments are stretched beyond their normal limits, they will tear or rupture like muscles, and they will lose their capacity to hold the back bones together. This will produce a fragile back that will be very susceptible to injury.

Ligaments are richly supplied with "sensory nerves" which may be damaged if the ligaments are torn. These nerves are responsible for the severe pain that accompanies a ligament injury. The pain may continue even after the ligament has healed.

Ligaments cannot repair themselves if they are completely torn. They can only be repaired surgically by removing torn sections and replacing them with other tissue. If ligaments are not repaired, joints will not operate properly, and pain and loss of function will result.

The most common source of ligament damage in the back comes from tearing or cracking of the annulus fibrosus, which leads to disc herniation.

It's important to be able to diagnose ligament damage. If it were missed, and treatment were directed only to bones, muscles, or discs, pain and loss of function would probably continue. Your ligaments may seem to be subtle components of your body's anatomy, but if they're damaged, they will make significant contributions to pain and discomfort.

6. NERVOUS SYSTEM

Your nervous system coordinates and controls responses to stimuli that affect your entire body. Because of the immense complexity of your nervous system, it's role in back problems is often neither appreciated nor completely understood. The nervous system is, however, involved not only with the cause and effect of bad backs, but also the psychological and physiological aspects of back problems.

This chapter describes how the major divisions of your nervous system are involved in back problems. It also discusses the type of nerve damage that commonly occurs with bad backs.

MAJOR DIVISIONS

The human nervous system is described and classified according to the function and purpose of the nerves it contains. Two major divisions exist; the central nervous system and the autonomic nervous system.

The central nervous system consists of your brain and spinal cord. It supervises and coordinates voluntary activity and provides control and direction over bodily movements and activities. The brain-directed central nervous system requires an act of will, or a mental calculation, involving thousands of messages that are received from all of your body's sensors.

The autonomic nervous system governs involuntary actions. It operates automatically to regulate breathing, heart action, movement of your intestines, vision, constriction and dilation of blood vessels, and glandular secretion.

The autonomic nervous system is divided functionally into the sympathetic and parasympathetic nervous systems. These two systems produce opposite effects in response to your body's needs, even though they both serve the same organs. The sympathetic nervous system is designed to speed things up, like making rapid adjustments in breathing and heartbeat during an emergency. The parasympathetic nervous system acts to slow things down and bring your body back to normal when danger is passed. The sympathetic nervous system acts as an accelerator, while the parasympathetic system acts as a brake.

When you experience unusual stress and tension, the sympathetic system stimulates your bodily functions to protect you. The effect on your body can be harmful if the sympathetic nervous system is constantly called into action because of the continued presence of stress. This is particularly true with the recurrence of painful muscle spasms. Eliminating the stress will allow the parasympathetic nervous system to bring your body back to a relaxed condition so that spasms can stop.

The nerves that make up your nervous system are also classified into two major groups according to their location in your body. The first group includes the nerves of the central nervous system that are found in the brain and spinal cord. The second group includes the peripheral nerves, so called because they serve numerous functions in the periphery of your body. Extending out from the spinal cord, through openings in the vertebrae, are 31 pairs of peripheral nerve roots. They transmit sensory impulses, including pain, from various parts of your body through the spinal cord to your brain. They also transmit motor impulses from the brain and spinal cord to the voluntary muscles. Most back pain comes when the peripheral nerves are irritated at the point where they leave the spinal cord.

Pain can come from deep within your body or the tips of your fingers. It can be triggered by injury or repeated stress. It's up to your nervous system to communicate and describe the nature of pain so proper treatment can be administered before nerve damage occurs.

NERVE DAMAGE

When nerves are pinched, they hurt. When a disc herniates through its outer covering into the spinal canal, one or more spinal nerve roots can get pinched against the bony vertebrae, causing intense back and leg pain. At other times, a nerve may be squeezed between two muscles that are in spasm. The pain from each of these two occurrences is quite similar and the inability to distinguish between them can lead to misdiagnosis and improper treatment.

When a nerve is compressed for an extended period, it stops transmitting pain signals because it dies. Nerves can, however, repair themselves by generating new fibres, but only after the killing force has been removed. Accordingly, proper diagnosis and appropriate treatment are essential for avoiding extensive nerve damage.

Destroying nerves is not a good way to eliminate pain as some people might believe. That's like killing the messenger for bringing bad news. Your nerves are needed to alert you to the dangers that pain represents. To obtain relief, you must attack the source of pain, not the system that transmits it.

7. PAIN

Back problems and chronic pain are constant companions. Pain is, in fact, the universal symptom of back disorders. Back pain is debilitating, costly, and difficult to eliminate. It is also communicative. It lets you know when psychological and physiological stress and tension have exceeded normal tolerance levels. Pain triggers unconscious reactions, which are intended to protect your bad back from additional damage. Pain is an aid to diagnosis, but it is also a threat to mental health.

This chapter describes the nature and effect of chronic pain. It also discusses the different ways in which pain is perceived.

CHRONIC PAIN

Sometimes back pain is acute, lasting for only a brief period of time. But for millions of people, back pain has become a chronic condition. It is the most common chronic-pain syndrome in America, accounting for more than 18 million physician-office visits each year. Chronic pain virtually takes over the body and becomes a way of life.

Chronic pain affects not only people with bad backs, but also those afflicted with cancer, disease, or other disabilities. People who suffer from chronic pain, regardless of the cause, share some common attributes. On the average, they have lived with their pain for seven years, undergone three to five major operations, and spent from $50,000 to $100,000 in medical bills. Because many doctors treat chronic pain as acute pain, their patients have taken a lot of drugs, including tranquilizers, muscle relaxants, painkillers, and other

38

narcotics. There is a 50-50 chance that people with chronic pain are addicted to drugs, alcohol, or both.

The amount of money people with serious, debilitating pain spend for analgesic drugs or surgical procedures, added to the amount of money lost to the Nation's economy because of time spent away from jobs, totals at least $10 *billion* each year. That's a lot of money, but doesn't include the $900 million that is spent each year for nonprescription pain pills, liniments, and other medications.

A noted psychiatrist once said, "God gave us pain to protect us from danger. It was never meant to be a disability". Unfortunately, for many people with serious back problems, pain has become a life-shattering disability.

Chronic pain comes from continued aggrevation of assorted bodily disturbances, including injuries, structural deformities, glandular imbalance, disease, herniated discs, or damaged muscles, tendons, or ligaments. The pain radiates from the site of the initial trauma to other areas of the body that have become abused through aggrevation or compensation.

Referred pain is a term used to describe chronic pain that has moved beyond the initial source of irritation. It is often considerably removed from where the pain first occurred, and is characterized by aching joints and muscles, local tenderness, and muscle spasms.

Lumbago is a term often used to describe chronic or recurring pain in the lumbar region of the back. It is a painful rheumatic condition that involves the muscles in the lower back.

Chronic pain develops when the initial pain symptoms have been relieved, but the original cause of pain remains. If adequate measures are not taken to prevent chronic pain from developing, it may cause more serious problems than those resulting from the initial trauma. If a herniated disc is causing pain, and if it is left unattended, subsequent nerve irritation and muscle spasms may create havoc for a major portion of the body. A cycle of chronic pain can develop that will be extremely difficult to stop.

Because of its subjective nature, chronic pain is very difficult to measure. It can only be assessed from descriptions given by one who is suffering. Accordingly, a clear perception of pain is critical for diagnosis and treatment.

PERCEPTION OF PAIN

The way the brain interprets incoming pain signals varies greatly from person to person. The intensity of the pain does not necessarily depend on the severity of the cause. That's why it's hard to understand back pain. The precipitating cause is often hard to identify and describe. What causes intense pain for one person may be considered inconsequential by another who is only slightly aggrieved. Because of the mysterious nature of back disorders, doctors are often unsympathetic toward, or even unprepared to treat the pain, let alone the cause.

The perception of pain can also be influenced by a person's family or by cultural factors. If other members of the family are unsympathetic toward pain, or if cultural mores discourage the expression of pain, a person with a bad back may in fact not perceive a high level of pain. On the other hand, in a less restrictive environment, the bad-back sufferer may perceive tremendous amounts of pain, some of which may be self-serving.

The fact that there is a wide variation in the way pain is perceived by different people, or by the same person at different times or under different circumstances, has provided one of the most important clues to the mysteries of pain. Researchers now suspect that there are mechanisms in the body, as well as in the brain, that can either alleviate pain or make it worse. It is also believed that these mechanisms operate totally without regard to the specific sources of pain.

Researchers also believe that perception of pain is influenced by controls in the brain that regulate anxiety, memory of past experiences, and suggestions. Such theories help explain individual differences in pain response, and show how the mind can play an important part in the perception of pain.

Not only is the mind involved in the perception of pain, but it also plays an important role in the development, continuation, and elimination of back problems. As the next chapter indicates, the mind affects those aspects of back disorders that are not readily apparent to either the doctor or the patient.

8. PSYCHE

Psyche is a general term used to describe your mind, mental capacity, psychological structure, or mentality. It is as important in the diagnosis and treatment of bad backs as vertebrae, discs, muscles, or nerves.

This chapter discusses some of the interrelationships between back problems and your psyche. Specific attention is given to stress and tension, psychosomatic problems, and enigmatic pain.

STRESS AND TENSION

Stress and tension are directly responsible for continued back pain. When you are anxious and under stress, your muscles become tense. Continued muscular contraction, resulting from stress and emotional tension, will close off blood vessels in your muscle tissues. This will prevent the vessels from carrying off waste products and supplying food and oxygen. When wastes build up, nerve endings become irritated, causing muscle spasm pain that is every bit as severe as that sustained from a traumatic injury.

Very few doctors believe emotional problems are the primary cause of back disorders. But doctors have found evidence suggesting that emotions play an important part in the severity of pain that is experienced. They have also found that the presence of emotional stress influences the treatment of bad backs.

The standard treatments for back pain—rest, hot showers and baths, whirlpool treatments, and massage—have a significant effect on the psyche as well as on sore and tender back muscles. Warm water, rest, and massage help people relax, and in turn relieve much

41

of the stress and strain on muscles. As muscles relax, normal blood flow is restored, and pain is reduced.

In many cases, weight loss and exercise will help alleviate bad-back problems. But if emotional stress is a precipitating factor, back problems will continue until the stress is eliminated. A supposedly effective exercise program may fail to serve its purpose if emotional stress continues to bring on muscular tension. Exercises that are designed to relax and strengthen muscles may be unable to overcome pervasive stress conditions. If stress is not recognized and dealt with, frustration will be directed toward the exercise program, which may then be erroneously discarded.

Weight loss is also affected by emotional stress. If loss of excess weight is due to stress instead of appropriate changes in dietary habits, weight gain may occur when stress is reduced. The effects of stress may mask bad eating habits, especially when weight is kept at desired levels.

The net effect of emotional stress and tension may be the rejection of needed exercise and the neglect of good dietary habits.

Sometimes stress is generated from within an individual rather than from some external source. In that case, the psyche becomes the focus of treatment rather than an adjunct element of the complaint.

PSYCHOSOMATIC PROBLEMS

If any physical ailment is primarily due to psychological stress, or if the reported pain is out of proportion to actual physical conditions, the disability is considered psychosomatic.

This does not mean that the pain is imaginary, or that the person who is suffering has a serious psychological problem. It does mean that psychological and not physiological problems are the precipitating cause of the disability.

Physicians are beginning to play closer attention to the psychological aspects of back pain. Specialists don't agree on what proportion of bad backs are essentially psychosomatic in origin, but almost all doctors agree that the way a person handles stress plays an important role in susceptibility to back pain.

People who are experiencing severe back pain become extremely resentful of others who suggest the existence of a psychosomatic problem. It is quite natural for one who has never been bothered by back pain to find it difficult to accept the dynamics of back disorders. Skeptics feel the only possible explanation for such mysterious, long-term, and limiting conditions is that they have to be imagined. Depending upon the relationship between the person in pain and the skeptic, the situation may bring on a wide range of new tensions and anxieties.

Husbands may be suspicious of wives who wish to refrain from sexual relations because of back pain. Employers may question an employee's job dedication when repeated requests are made to take time out during the day to lie down. More seriously, however, a doctor may discount as psychosomatic the complaints of a patient who is also a close friend. Withholding corrective treatment may compound the back problems, and the psychosomatic diagnosis may end a friendship.

ENIGMATIC PAIN

One of the most frustrating aspects of a bad back is the mysterious and vague nature of the ailment. You may go for three or four days in intense pain and then suddenly have a good day with little or no pain. Perhaps a protruding disc retracted and no longer pressed on a spinal nerve. Perhaps your pain of previous days was residual pain, resulting from a much earlier problem, such as a sprain or strain that subsequently healed.

What you do on the day your pain goes away will have a significant effect on what happens in the days ahead. Many people feel elated when their pain finally disappears. They scurry about doing many things they were previously unable to do, and they will probably do too much. A day or two later, pain may return, even more severe than before. Instead of letting nerves and muscles recuperate on a pain-free day, the bad-back victim forces them to work even harder than before.

The psychological effects of enigmatic pain may be devastating. Your feeling of elation on one day can be replaced with a feeling of despair the next. The shift in mood from elation to depression is usually very dramatic. The stress that accompanies depression will aggrevate the nerves and muscles in your back, and the pain cycle will be off and running again.

On another occasion, you may decide to follow your doctor's ,recommendation to rest on a pain-free day. Your day of rest may be spent on a heating pad in quiet anticipation of a second pain-free day that will surely follow. But for some unknown reason, pain returns and there is no second good day. You may become very frustrated when a conscientious attempt to take corrective action is repaid with additional pain. Frustration may then lead to depression and stress, resulting in additional muscle tension and pain.

A chronic back problem can be characterized by wildly fluxuating days of pain and relief. Changes in the weather, temperature shifts, or variations in barometric pressure can induce pain in weakened muscles. Bodily changes, such as menstrual periods, can also cause back-pain to reappear. Extraneous life situations, not immediately apparent to you or others, can produce enough tension to induce pain. The vacillating, uncertain nature of back pain can bring on additional stress and tension, resulting in more pain.

It is the enigmatic nature of back pain that can be so devastating to your psyche. Repeated bombardment will increase emotional stress and tension and cause additional problems for your already weakened back. And if back pain wasn't enough, additional aggrevation can come from the problems of aging as the next chapter points out.

9. AGE CRISES

Men and women who suffer serious back problems usually do so when they are in their late thirties and early forties. This is the period in life when many people are already facing other problems, including the crises of aging. The combination of bad-back problems and midlife crises can be devastating for some and strengthening for others.

This chapter discusses the nature and consequences of problems that are unique to a period in life when back difficulties tend to materialize.

MIDLIFE PROBLEMS

The midlife decade is generally identified as being between the ages of 35 and 45. The way people respond to the stress of this period can vary as much as the amount of stress they are under. During these years, there is a significant increase in the incidence of alcoholism, hypochondria, and obesity, all of which are associated with depression. Sexual problems, if they existed before, become worse. The divorce rate increases. Career changes also occur with increased frequency. For many men and women, this can be a tumultous period.

Men in particular have a difficult time in dealing with health problems at this stage in life. A man's psyche can take a real beating if he begins to suffer back problems while trying to cope with a midlife crisis. He probably has already begun to realize he does not have the control he once had over his body. He can't run as fast or work as hard. His recreational pursuits may have changed as his wealth increased and his family grew. He may spend more time with his family and friends in sedentary activities instead of in athletic games with his peers. Like so many others, he may continue to eat as voraciously as he did 10 years earlier, even though he is exercising less. Physically, he has let himself deteriorate, he knows it, and it causes him concern.

As he enters his forties, a man becomes acutely aware of the first signs of aging. He realizes he is on the downhill side of life and has passed the midway point in his race with death.

During his forties, a man's children also change. They become more independent, displaying the character their father helped to build. Depending on a man's expectations, he may be pleased or distressed by the directions his children take. If he is distressed, the resulting conflicts and tension may bring on additional stress that may be hard for him to cope with.

As a man's children become less dependent, he finds the reverse is true of his parents. He must now deal with the death or senility of those he loves and once looked up to. At a time when he seeks new horizons, his parents make increasing demands on him. As his children leave home, their places are often taken by his or his wife's parents.

All in all, the midlife decade can be pretty traumatic for many people. The prevailing stresses of the period can precipitate, aggrevate, or be influenced by back problems. Both men and women are susceptible to the combined effects of age crises and bad backs.

EFFECTS OF THE BAD BACK

Now comes the bad back. It could be aggrevated by a man's physical condition or the episodic stresses of the midlife decade. He may try to regain some of the athletic ability he once had, only to be stopped by back pain. Fighting fears of waning sexual virility, he may seek more frequent and active sexual encounters. Each occurrence may prove painful and frustrating if his back pain is severe.

In essence, a bad back, occurring during a midlife crisis, may signify to a man the start of physical deterioration that is catapulting him towards death. The normal life stresses of this period may aggrevate his physical condition as already taxed muscles and nerves cope with added damage caused by the bruising of his psyche. The depression all of this causes tends to keep the cycle of stress and pain running. Rehabilitation is difficult because treatment must be directed to psychological as well as physiological factors.

HUSBAND-WIFE RELATIONSHIPS

The role of wives in this midlife period cannot be overlooked. If both husband and wife can live with his changing personality, including his reaction to back problems, their marital relationship will probably remain strong. But the wife is also experiencing change. For years she has had to satisfy the needs of her children. Now that her children are becoming independent and leaving home, she begins to seek new forms of self-expression. An overweight, depressed husband with a bad back may be an albatross around her neck, keeping her from gaining the independence she now seeks. Resentment toward her husband may lead to fewer sexual encounters, which for him may compound his feelings of inadequacy. A split between them may widen into a chasm.

Women who experience back problems during this midlife decade also face a difficult period of adjustment. This is especially true for their relationships with their husbands. A husband who is denied lovemaking by his pain-ridden wife, and who at the same time must assume the role of mother and homemaker, may develop intense feelings of hostility. The wife finds the hostility difficult to cope with, because she doesn't know if it is directed toward her or her bad-back condition. Her body and her outlook on life are both changing as much as her husband's. Even though the roles of husbands and wives are generally quite different, the difficulties they experience, tend to be shared between them.

Back problems tend to aggrevate life crises for both husbands and wives. This is because of the long-term, pervasive, and enigmatic nature of back pain, and the significance of the events occurring at the time in people's lives when back problems most commonly occur. Some people are able to get through this period unscathed. Others experience just enough stress to unnecessarily prolong their back problems. Unfortunately, many others are unable to cope with the combination of pain and stress, and their marriage, employment, and interpersonal relationships may all be devastated.

10. SUMMARY OF PART I

Back problems are very complex because of the almost unbelievable number of factors that are involved. In order for you to overcome your bad back, you must know and understand everything you can about the way your back is put together. You must also understand the impact that social and psychological influences have on the nature and extent of back problems.

Part I contains essential information about the structure and function of the back, including physiological and psychological elements of the body that are affected when back problems occur. It describes the nature and arrangement of the spinal column and its supporting elements. It explains how bones grow and repair themselves, and it describes three of the many bone-related problems that can affect your back. It also describes the structure of the intervertebral discs as well as the nature and cause of disc problems. It describes the nature and function of back muscles, and the need for maintaining proper muscle tone. Muscle damage and muscle spasms are also discussed.

Part I also identifies the most important ligaments in the back and describes what can happen when they are damaged. It describes the major divisions of the nervous system and the types of nerve damage that accompanies a bad back. It also describes the nature of chronic pain, which is a frequent companion to bad backs. The way pain is perceived is also discussed.

Part I describes some aspects of bad backs that directly affect a person's psychological condition. Specific attention is given to stress and tension, psychosomatic problems, and enigmatic pain. Finally,

Part I discusses the nature and consequence of problems that are unique to a period in life when back problems tend to materialize.

PART II

COPING WITH LIFE
SITUATIONS

11. LIVING, NOT GIVING UP

Some people with bad backs have been told by their doctors and others that theirs is a condition they will just have to live with. Furthermore, they have been told they will have to learn to accept pain, disability, and restricted activity as a way of life. Some people believe this even though no one told them so.

It's sad, but this misguided advice has been given in far too many cases. You don't have to give in to your back problems, because there are ways of escaping pain and disability. If you've been told otherwise, it's just not true, unless you're suffering a terminal illness. You can live with a bad back without surrendering to it. In fact, you should take the offensive and overcome your bad back..

The chapters in Part II identify and describe some major problems of daily living that are encountered by people with bad backs. Several suggestions for eliminating those problems are also presented. As the following list illustrates, the range of subject matter in each chapter is pretty broad.

A General Approach
Back Pain and Work
Sex
Marriage and Family
Social Life
Doctors
Drugs and Alcohol
Standing, Lifting, Sitting, Sleeping
Depression and Positive Attitudes

The suggestions presented in Part II are meant to complement the care given by licensed professionals, not replace it. Direct your questions to the professionals, but also give consideration to the thoughts of those who have experienced back problems and lived through many of the concerns discussed in these chapters. By gathering as much information as possible, you will be well on your way toward overcoming your bad back.

The next chapter describes some general strategies for coping with life situations when disabled by a bad back.

12. A GENERAL APPROACH

Everyone who experiences back pain, regardless of the cause, can take some common measures to hasten recovery. These are simple steps, designed to provide relief from pain and guide the recovery process. Some involve immediate action, while others are concerned with long-term care.

This chapter discusses procedures that should be followed at the onset of back problems. It also suggests ways of dealing with back problems that last for long periods. Finally, it suggests several specific courses of action that can be very helpful in a wide variety of situations.

FIRST AID

Many back problems come on suddenly as a result of injury or the aggrevation of hereditary defects. Other problems, stemming from tumors, infections, hormonal changes, or chronic strain, may develop over extended periods of time. In either case, pain and other symptoms may appear without warning, resulting in unexpected disability.

It seems strange, but many people don't think their condition is serious when back pain first strikes. Unfortunately, the notion that back pain will somehow vanish can be very harmful. It postpones action that could not only bring about an early solution, but also prevent serious problems that probably will appear later. If the symptoms are ignored, the back will continue to hurt, or the pain will temporarily disappear, only to come back again when least expected.

There are a number of immediate steps you should take regardless of whether a doctor is called later or not. The first thing you should do is lie down and rest. If your pain is serious, muscles and nerves are obviously involved, and there is a good chance a bad disc might also be. Lying down will bring immediate relief, allowing muscles to relax while reducing pressure on weakened discs. Rest will also help prevent further damage to affected areas.

The second step involves the use of medications. A nonprescription pain remedy like aspirin can relieve pain and in many cases the tension that goes with it. Tranquilizers or muscle relaxants prescribed by your doctor may be helpful if they don't become habit forming. If the condition is very serious, your doctor might prescribe more powerful medication.

A third step might involve hot baths or whirlpool treatments, which tend to reduce tension and ease aching muscles. A hot shower may be better for you since sitting in a bath tub could place additional pressure on already-weakened discs and sore muscles. The body movement required for getting in and out of a bathtub might also add to existing muscle strain.

Back pain creates uncertainty and apprehension when people begin to think about surgery and prolonged disability. Added nervousness and tension from any source will add significantly to the amount of pain you will experience. That's why it's very important to relax as soon as possible following an attack of back pain.

If extended disability is anticipated or expected, a number of other strategies become very useful.

KEEP A DIARY

You can become an expert on your back condition by keeping a chronological record of everything that happens to you. The events of every day should be entered—the good as well as the bad. You should write down what you did and how you felt while doing it. Document changes in the weather, since they can significantly affect the way you feel. Describe the medications you take and the effects they have. Keep a record of your weight, describe the exercises you are able to perform, and make note of any physical limitations you experience.

After taking good care of yourself for three or four weeks, you may feel your back has not improved at all. A review of your diary should prove otherwise. The psychological lift that comes with discovering progress will do wonders for you.

If no progress is evident, or if you are experiencing more pain and less mobility, consult your doctor immediately. Your diary will provide documented evidence of all that has happened to you. It will be immensely beneficial to your doctor in developing or modifying your treatment plan.

If possible, extend your diary backwards in time. Try to identify significant events that may have caused your back problems. You may have suffered an injury, added extra body weight, or begun a prolonged period of stress. The more you learn about the past, the more you will know about the present and what to expect in the future.

Keeping an accurate chronology of events is very important in the care and treatment of your bad back. But the way you spend your time is just as important.

USE YOUR TIME WISELY

Time can be your best friend or worst enemy when trying to overcome a bad back. The way you use your time for healing will play a significant part in your overall treatment program. You may, for example, decide to rest in bed for a week to let your back heal. But it is possible for your pain and discomfort to be as bad at the end of the week as they were at the beginning. If they are, you may feel the week was wasted and vow not to stay down again. Your frustration may lead you to work twice as hard, trying to catch up on what you feel you've lost.

But maybe you should have taken two weeks instead of one. It's foolish to think you can't take as much time as you need to let your back heal. That's like saying you'll only use a limited amount of water to save your burning house. If more time is needed, either be ready to take it, or adjust your life to an extended period of costly pain and inconvenience.

You should plan to make good use of any time you set aside for healing. Reading about the nature and treatment of bad backs can be very helpful, especially if you discover a program of diet and mild exercise that you will enjoy. You may also discover from your reading that you are worse off than you had imagined. Your new knowledge should prompt you to make an appointment with a back specialist.

Plans should also be made for the time following rest periods. Think of new ways of doing normal activities at home or at work. Eliminate activities that produce stress and tension or cause pain in your back.

Look to the future. Nothing is lost from a rest period except time. It's gone, you can't get it back, and you can't double up on the time remaining by doing twice as much as before. Assess your position realistically, and concentrate on your next moves for overcoming your bad back. If a period of rest didn't seem to help, maybe something else will. Consult your doctor or someone who specializes in back problems. Start an exercise or diet program. Schedule a trip to the library to find out more about your condition. Be careful, but be aggressive. Take the offensive in dealing with your bad back, and make good use of whatever time you have.

COURSES OF ACTION

There are many things you can and should do to overcome bad-back problems. As a start, you can apply the following suggestions to almost every situation in which you find yourself, whether at work, in your home, or in a variety of social settings. Later in this book, other suggestions are offered for dealing with specific sets of circumstances.

Don't Delay. Take time off and rest before you have to go to a hospital for treatment, or before irreparable damage is done to your back. Immediate bed rest can reduce pressure on a slightly herniated disc, allowing it to retract into the intervertebral space where it belongs. On the other hand, continued pressure from standing and working may cause the disc to protrude further into the spinal canal where it will press against a nerve, increasing pain and causing subsequent nerve damage. Continued herniation may reduce elasticity of a disc, leaving it vulnerable to subsequent problems.

Overworked or weakened muscles also need rest. Without it, they may fail to support the back when support is needed.

Share Your Knowledge. Have a straightforward talk with your spouse, employer, fellow workers, and children. Tell them everything you have learned about your back problems, especially your requirements for getting better. Don't withhold anything from those whose expectations you hope to meet. If you don't tell them, they may draw their own conclusions—many of which may be wrong. If the facts are known, others will probably do what they can to help you.

Avoid Deadlines. Don't set a specific deadline for overcoming your back problems. Failure to meet a firm deadline could have a devastating effect on your attitude. Those who know of your deadline may also be disappointed if you don't achieve your goal.

So many complicated factors are associated with back pain that it is almost impossible to set a deadline for one or more of them to be eliminated. The best you can do is take one day at a time and try to improve your condition from one day to the next. Without the pressure of a deadline, you should begin to feel better in much less time.

Prepare For The Worst. Think of the worst possible thing that could happen to you at your job or at home because of your bad back. It could mean you will be fired, because you can no longer do the work that is expected of you. It could also mean your marriage will suffer or your family will be seriously disrupted. Write down all of your worst fears, and describe how you would manage if such catastrophic events were to come true.

If you prepare for the worst, you will find your fears get smaller. Some even disappear. You can avoid a lot of pain-provoking stress and anxiety by addressing your fears head-on. On the other hand, if you spend your time worrying, the resulting stress and tension will play havoc with sore muscles and nerves, and your back will get worse instead of better.

Listen To Others. If people ask, tell them what you are doing to eliminate your back problems, and ask that they bear with you during difficult periods. Some people will not understand no matter what you say or how you say it. Others may provide helpful suggestions you never thought of before.

Suggestions on how to take care of your back may come from your spouse, doctor, friends, fellow workers, or employer. You may initially reject their suggestions if you feel they are intruding. Such reactions are natural, but they may interfere with your recovery.

As long as your back hurts and others know it, you will be given suggestions on how to get better. If a suggestion sounds reasonable (and even if it doesn't) give it consideration and pursue it. The back is a mysterious apparatus, and the cure of a bad back can take many forms. Don't discard a single suggestion no matter how outlandish it may sound or how suspect you are of the motivation behind it. Thank the one who gave it to you, honestly say you will look into it, scrutinize it closely, accept or reject it, and then tell the one who gave it to you what you decided and why. Your life may become a lot easier if you follow these simple steps. You may learn more about your back, and you may win new friends and keep those you already have.

Look Around You. When you are suffering pain every day, you probably tend to focus on yourself even though you know others may hurt more. In one sense, you are being selfish, but more importantly, you may be missing something. Look around you at people who are able to handle pain that is equal to or worse than yours. Some people may be going to pain clinics to learn about pain and how to conquer it. Others may have developed a reservoir of faith that sustains them. Whatever they are doing may work for you as well. Direct your attention away from your own misery, and see if others can show you the way to overcome your bad back.

Sometimes, the unique nature of a situation requires a slightly different strategy. The next chapter, as an example, focuses on the stresses of the work environment. Subsequent chapters deal with other life situations that present special difficulties for bad back sufferers.

13. BACK PAIN AND WORK

People work in homes and factories, on farms and in cities, and in a wide variety of occupations and settings. They are either self-employed, or they look to others for their employment. Regardless of their work environment, everyone exerts some form of sustained physical and mental activity to accomplish work objectives.

People with bad backs, however, generally find it difficult to meet those work objectives. As their output diminishes, pain-provoking stress and tension build up over a real or perceived loss of income or termination of employment.

This chapter identifies and describes some of the stress and tension that is characteristically present in work environments. It also provides suggestions for coping with work-related stress that is precipitated by bad-back problems.

WORK RELATED STRESS

Rest is one of the best remedies for back pain. Lying down for an extended period of time allows sore muscles to heal, reduces pressure on discs, and alleviates pain.

Unfortunately, people cannot always quit what they are doing to take time out for rest. Parents have families that need their attention. Employers have job requirements that must be fulfilled. Production deadlines must be met. The rest of the world will not slow down or stop no matter how bad a person's back may be.

A work environment can produce tremendous amounts of pain-aggrevating stress for people with bad backs. Three of the most common types of stress situations are listed here.

Physical Demands. People with bad backs may be unable to meet the physical requirements of their jobs, whether self-imposed or part of essential job requirements. Parents may find it impossible to lift children or complete normal household tasks. Office workers and executives may be unable to sit at their desks for extended periods of time. Farmers, truck drivers, or those in similar occupations may be unable to operate heavy equipment. Even the simplest physical tasks may prove difficult for those who are handicapped by back pain.

Conscientious employees who are unable to meet the physical demands of their jobs may become extremely frustrated. If they push themselves to do the best they can, they may aggrevate their condition and be in worse shape than when their back pain first started. Their back problems, if precipitated by the physical demands of their jobs, may get worse just from going to work.

Feelings of Failure The inability to complete even the simplest work tasks because of back pain can be extremely stress-provoking for most employees. They may become defensive about their work, thinking that fellow workers are being critical of their efforts. They begin to experience feelings of failure and think others are accusing them of "goldbricking".

Stress builds in two ways. First, the individual in pain feels frustrated at not being able to perform normal job tasks. Second, the real or imagined criticism of fellow workers becomes difficult to cope with when aggrevated by performance frustrations and pain. It is not uncommon for people who are under such stress to feel they have failed their employers, their fellow workers, and themselves.

Unsuccessful Attempts. One of the most devastating situations bad-back sufferers can encounter follows a period of rest from their jobs. A sick leave may have been granted in an attempt to correct a bad back and eliminate pain. If the rest period is successful, the person may return to work in good condition, able to perform as before. But sometimes the pain at the end of the rest period is as bad as at the beginning.

If the rest period is unproductive, a tremendous amount of stress can build when work activities are resumed. Fellow workers will inquire about the rest and wonder why the back still hurts. They know that if a person goes to bed with a cold, the cold will probably go away. It's hard for many people to understand that a bad back may have been too far along for bed rest to cure it. Those who still hurt wish they could say they felt better, but their pain is too obvious to others. They feel their rest period was a waste of time, and they feel guilty for having taken it. With their feelings of guilt come tension, stress, and more pain. Hesitant to ask for another rest period, the person with the bad back works twice as hard to catch up on missed work. This extra activity will probably cause additional damage to already affected areas.

WORK GUIDELINES

The stress of hanging on to your job can be tremendous, especially if you feel your bad back might cause you to lose it. As a general course of action, you should take time to analyze the nature and extent of the stress you are under. Discover those things that are bothering you so you can deal with them in an effective manner. Beyond that, there are several other steps you can take to make your work environment more tolerable. Three suggestions are provided here.

Offer Alternatives. Identify those things that are hard for you to do and should be eliminated from your day-to-day activities. Offer to substitute less painful tasks that would still allow you to stay productive. Make it clear you are doing your best to contribute in whatever way you can. But also make it clear you are in pain and can't substitute one hard task for another if it brings on the same problems. Emphasize the temporary nature of the change and your desire to be back at your old job as soon as you can.

Sometimes you can change your time schedule. Start earlier in the day, work later, and take more time to rest. You might also be able to cut down the number of hours you work each day by working weekends.

If you try in good faith to do as much as you can, an understanding employer will try to accomodate your needs.

Explain Medications. If you are taking a muscle-relaxing drug and a painkiller at the same time, the combination can cause you to feel drunk or half asleep. Anything that has a tranquilizing effect will probably affect your ability to work. Explain this to your employer and your fellow workers, especially if you're working near heavy machinery. If your medications make it difficult for you to concentrate on traffic, don't hesitate to ask someone to do your driving for you.

If you need medication, don't try to hide the fact. Others will see you are not functioning 100 percent. If they know why you are using medications, they won't make wild guesses about your erratic behavior.

Alter Your Work Habits. To avoid continued aggrevation of your back, you should try to keep one foot raised while you're sitting or standing. Resting one foot on a stool or bottom desk drawer will reduce the curves in your back and decrease stress on your interverte-bral discs. Besides giving you some relief, the practice has historical precedence. The foot rail found in saloons was designed as a comfort for those who stood at the bar for long periods of time.

Take a cot to work, and lie down when you can. Most camping supply stores carry cots that fold easily and store in small spaces. Find an out-of-the-way place where you can set up your cot during your lunch break. Using it will help in several ways. First, getting off your feet or out of a sitting position will relieve sore muscles and reduce pressure on discs and nerves. Second, a midday rest will reduce the stress and tension of your job. You could also help your diet by spending your lunch period on a cot instead of going out for something to eat.

A few changes in work habits may be all that's necessary to alleviate a major source of pain-provoking stress and tension.

14. SEX

Most people can continue to enjoy healthy sexual activities even if they are experiencing serious back pain. To do so, however, may require some adjustments in sexual behavior and attitudes.

This chapter discusses some of the problems people encounter when they try to modify their sexual activity to accomodate continued back problems. It also provides suggestions for resolving those problems.

SEXUAL ADJUSTMENTS

Sexual activity is possible no matter how serious the back problems may be. It is also desirable, because it helps to stabilize a marriage and release emotional and physical tension. The release of tension is especially good for a bad back, but so is the physical activity involved in sex.

Prior to the occurrence of back problems, sexual relations may have been active and vigorous. But with one partner in pain, both must learn to be tender and gentle and yet sexually stimulating.

Sexual activity will not, by itself, inflict permanent damage to a bad back. The problem lies in finding some way to physically and emotionally satisfy both the person in pain and the healthy partner. A number of techniques may be used if they satisfy both partners and are not offensive to either one.

Neither partner should ignore or discount existing back pain in anticipation of normal sexual relations in the future. It must be clearly understood that back pain can recur, and that adjustment to sexual relations may be long-term in nature. If the partners totally withdraw from each other instead of accommodating to their immediate problems, they may establish an antagonistic relationship that could be difficult to overcome. The partners must face their new situation head-on without losing the warmth, tenderness, and excitement that characterized their relationship before the back problems began.

Back pain is not easy to escape while having sex. In the most common position of sexual intercourse, with the man face-to-face above the woman, the greatest amount of movement for the man alternates the position of the spine from humpback to swayback. This requires movement of the small of the back at the L4-L5 level, which is the site of most back problems. A man with a bad back can aggrevate a herniated disc or unstable vertebra when he moves forward, or he can painfully stretch his sciatic nerve when he pulls back. A woman with a bad back may find the weight of her partner, his thrusts, and other bodily movements to be extremely painful.

The principles of sensible back care should be followed in sexual intercourse as with every other physical activity. It is better to abstain if back pain is severe. When sexual relations are resumed, they should be done so as not to aggrevate painful conditions. This may require some adjustments in a couple's normal pattern of sexual behavior.

The key to good sex is not found in a variety of positions or movements, however. Love, tenderness, and the desire to please are the most important factors. The person suffering from back pain can have an active and pleasant sex life as long as a sympathetic and understanding partner is willing to help.

Earlier sexual behavior can be restored when pain and back problems are gone. In the meantime, the partners should try to discover movements that avoid pain, but still bring pleasure. Sometimes moderation is the only adjustment that needs to be made.

Some people fall into a pattern of sexual behavior that was appropriate when one partner was in pain, and they find it difficult to change that behavior after the back has healed. Stress and tension remain, and sexual difficulties are accentuated. For others, the episode of pain brought them closer together. There is now more variety, more tenderness, and more of a sense of giving in their relationship.

PROBLEMS WITH ORGASM

Orgasm is the physical and emotional climax of a sexual act. It is normally a pleasant and exciting sensation, but it can be painful and frightening for a person with a bad back.

Difficulties arise because nerves in the genital area connect to the spinal cord in the region of the lower back. Thus, orgasm can cause intense pain when already weakened nerves suffer additional irritation. A person with a bad back may at the same time experience the pleasures of orgasm and the torment of a muscle spasm. To know what to do in that situation requires a great deal of patience, understanding, love, and gentleness.

The inability to reach orgasm because of psychological reasons or because of impotence can constitute a serious marital problem for either partner. But the inability to reach orgasm because of the presence of intense pain can be even more frustrating. Stress occurs when the healthy partner must stop because of the other person's pain. The resulting frustration can turn to anger, rejection, or hostility.

Hostility should not be directed to the person with the bad back, nor should the one with the bad back feel guilty. Sometimes, one partner, wracked with spasms and pain, may allow the healthy partner to continue to orgasm. That's nonsense, and it could aggrevate existing back problems. If pain gets bad, sexual relations should stop. If orgasm is close, it can happen in other ways that won't cause so much pain.

The frustrations surrounding orgasm must be dealt with openly and directly by both partners to avoid irrepairable damage to their relationship.

PSYCHOLOGICAL FACTORS

Many people find that sexual activity relieves stress and produces a feeling of calm and satisfaction, especially if orgasm is reached. It is probably true in most marriages that the act of sexual intercourse has been performed as much for enjoyment as for love of the partner. But seeking sex for personal satisfaction with no regard for the pain and agony of the partner can be devastating. The one with a bad back may be worse off because of sexual activity, and the guilt of exploitation may create additional stress for the one who selfishly sought satisfaction of sexual desires.

Sometimes, fear of recurring disc pain prevents men from getting an erection. Women, being just as frightened, can become frigid. In most cases, there is nothing physiologically wrong with either partner. They are merely reacting psychologically to the presence or threat of pain. Doctors who have studied the sexual activity of men who have back problems find that for each case of organic impotence, there are at least nine cases of psychological impotence.

There are, however, other back-related factors that can influence sexual activity. Back surgery may injure essential nerves, diminishing the ability to achieve satisfactory sexual relationships. Drugs, taken to relieve pain or to relax muscles, may also have negative effects on the sex act by causing impotency or the inability to be stimulated to orgasm. These should be considered when dealing with suspected impotence or frigidity.

DEALING WITH SEXUAL PROBLEMS

If either you or your partner are experiencing a significant amount of pain, and if sex is to be avoided, the attitude the healthy partner must develop is critical.

Many people do not find it difficult to abstain from sex. Priests take vows of celibacy as part of their religious committment. But they don't find themselves face-to-face with a loving, warm body each night. It is very difficult to get in bed and to reach out to touch your partner, to feel that soft, warm body next to yours, and not be able to make love.

It helps in breaking most bad habits, or in changing established behavioral patterns, if you discount the satisfaction the act has given. You may have given up smoking or some other habit by believing it was bad and should not be done. But you don't do that with sex. You cannot develop negative attitudes toward your partner as a way of lessening your desire for sex. You need to remain loving, warm, and affectionate. You must somehow submerge your need and desire for sex, while at the same time maintain your positive feelings toward the one with whom you cannot make love. This is not an easy task if it goes on for several months, nor are there common strategies for coping with the problems it brings.

If your back hurts, you will not be able to participate in or enjoy sex as if your back was free of pain. But most of the sexual problems you will encounter will be psychological and not physical. There is always the fear you will hurt yourself if you engage in sexual activity. If your partner has a bad back, you may abstain out of fear of causing additional pain and disability.

Sexual activity can be made more pleasurable if pain and discomfort are reduced before going to bed. Hot baths, back rubs, or the use of analgesics can all help. The same procedures can be used after sexual relations. Back rubs and massage can reduce the muscle spasms that may accompany orgasm.

Most people find it difficult to talk about problems of sex. If communication is lacking, a reason for abstaining may sound more like an excuse. Personal feelings and problems should be openly discussed so that neither you nor your partner develops ill feelings toward the other. If you remember that the key to a good sexual relationship lies in love, tenderness, and the desire to please, you will be able to talk about and discover sexual activities that will not be pain producing.

Masturbation may arise as one alternative to an unfulfilled sex life. Depending on your attitudes, this act may be unacceptable to you even though it may relieve the stress and frustration that abstinence brings. Consider it carefully and talk about it openly with your partner. Both of you may feel your sex life is unsatisfactory without knowing how to change it. Express and share your frustrations. If masturbation is seen as an alternative, and one or the other engages in it to reach orgasm, feelings of guilt or dissatisfaction may still be present. Such feelings must be shared and dealt with by both partners.

You need not experience any sexual difficulties because of a lack of information. Several self-help books are available in libraries and bookstores, and many social service agencies, colleges and universities, and medical clinics provide counseling and guidance in the area of sexual relations. If stress and tension exist because of sexual problems, you should seek help and additional information as aggressively as you do for the physical problems in your back.

Maintaining a healthy and fulfilling sex life is not an easy task for people who are suffering back pain and disability. Since both physical and psychological difficulties are involved, problem solving becomes very complex. Both partners must be willing to adopt new behaviors in order for marital stress and tension to be avoided.

15. MARRIAGE AND FAMILY

Bad-back problems can make life miserable for others besides the one who is afflicted, especially spouses and other family members. Stress and tension caused by back problems can cause disharmony in the family, or they can serve as catalysts that brings everyone closer together.

This chapter discusses the stress that families experience when one member has a bad back. It also discusses family reactions to that stress and provides suggestions for coping with problems that occur.

MARITAL STRESS

Marriage is a sharing experience. When one partner can no longer share in the responsibilities or obligations of marriage because of back problems, a disproportionate load is passed to the healthy partner. A wife or husband may have to take another job to augment the income a disabled mate can no longer provide. A husband may have to assume the duties of motherhood in addition to being a father. A working mother may have to take on additional household responsibilities that her pain-ridden husband previously shared.

If neither spouse has ever experienced debilitating pain, they may at first become suspicious or resentful of the one who can no longer share the load. Healthy partners may be puzzled at the way their mate behaves and they may become impatient with the prolonged nature of the apparent ailment. They may feel their partner is malingering and the pain is imagined. The ensuing doubt and resentment will create stress for both partners.

The presence of pain can also affect marital obligations. One parent may have to go alone to a school event, party, church function, or social gathering because the spouse is home in bed with a bad back. A fine line exists between an excuse and a justified reason for not attending an event that affects both marriage partners. Unless the marriage is built on trust and honesty, one-parent participation may lead to skepticism, anger, or other problems.

GIVERS AND TAKERS

The way people relate to others will have a significant effect on the happiness of the family. In general, people either give assistance to others, or they take all the help they can get. And there are, of course, many people between the two extremes.

People who give of themselves tend to help others who are in difficulty, want, or distress. Givers are quite common. They are the first to bring a meal, offer rides, or provide other help. Some people give of themselves compulsively. They feel a day is not complete unless they have extended a helping hand to someone else. Most parents are givers, especially toward their children. Some givers enjoy feelings of authority or dominance in their giving. They tend not to stay down when they are ill or disabled, feeling inability to care for themselves is a sign of weakness. They will give, but they will not readily accept care and attention from others.

Takers are quite the opposite of givers. When they are sick or disabled, they are quick to look elsewhere for help. They are very dependent upon the solicitous attitude of others. Because takers tend to receive more than they give, they are sometimes accused of being malingerers or hypochondriacs. It is difficult for takers to extend a helping hand to others, because they are so totally dependent upon the giving of other people. In American society, this behavior among adults is generally not acceptable.

In a family situation, one or both parents tend to be givers. It is not unusual, however, for one spouse to be a giver and the other a taker, without regard to sex. Children, especially if they are teenagers or younger, tend to be takers, because they generally don't have the means to provide for themselves and others as well. As children grow older and more independent, they begin to change from taking to giving.

The status of giving and taking within a family can be altered significantly when back problems strike one or more parents. A mother who is used to serving the needs of those around her may suddenly find herself completely incapacitated. A father who is helplessly flat on his back in bed may no longer feel he is the dominant member of the family. Both parents will be frustrated by their inability to satisfy the needs of those they feel depend on them. They will also be frustrated when others try to help them, since that will accentuate their dependency.

Many parents don't like to become dependent on other members of the family, particularly their children. A mother is often unwilling to relinquish her kitchen to her children or her husband. Many parents hesitate to ask their children to cook meals, wash clothes, or clean house, especially when they lack confidence in their children's abilities.

Children find their parents' back problems equally frustrating. Those who have had to depend on their parents find it difficult to learn new skills that are suddenly thrust upon them. Some children resent it; others may welcome the chance to become independent and helpful. Children may become frustrated and angry if they are stiffled by a giving parent who will neither relinquish authority, nor graciously accept giving behavior from a child.

RESENTMENT

Frustrations that develop within a family because of back problems can lead to resentment that will manifest itself in at least two ways.

Resentment can come from feeling that the one who complains of back problems is really malingering. Those who are doing the work may feel the bad back is not as bad as the afflicted one would like to have others believe. This kind of resentment can be alleviated if the back condition has been carefully studied and explained to every family member. If resentment still exists after the facts have been presented, it probably comes from selfish reasons, and there is little that can be done to eliminate it.

The second kind of resentment comes from the way people with bad backs take care of themselves. Most people do not like to see another person afflicted with pain. They are more than willing to help, but they expect something in return. Those who provide help to someone in need expect the recipient to be working just as hard at getting better as they are as providing care. If a person has been recuperating for a long time, and has been waited on regularly, a lot of good feeling can be destroyed if they try to do something that is far beyond their capabilities, especially if it threatens their back condition. Resentment may build in the giver because the taker is doing senseless things to prolong a bad-back problem. Most people will generally want to help another, but they will resent it deeply if they feel the taker is not working equally as hard at overcoming their bad back.

FAMILY GUIDELINES

If you're suffering from a bad back, be gracious and accept the helping hand of others, but don't take an arm and a leg as well by making unreasonable demands. Don't do senseless things that will prolong your condition and tax the patience of those who are trying to help you. Accept their care and return their kindness when they are in need.

Discuss your condition with other family members. Tell them why you hurt and what you have to do to get better. Describe your limitations. Answer questions or suggest other sources of information. If every member of the family knows what your problems are, less friction, stress, or tension will exist.

Set priorities within the family. If your children are active and would like you to attend their events, ask them to help you set priorities for what you can and cannot attend. Sometimes they may not want you in attendance. Find out what's important and work out a schedule.

If you're a working spouse with a bad back, you should also set some priorities. You are not being fair to yourself, or to your family, if you thoroughly exhaust yourself on the job and then have no time to give to your spouse or your children. Only an extremely demanding work situation could so captivate you that you cannot find time for your family. But if that's the case, be sure your family knows and understands the situation.

Be a diplomat and make concessions if necessary. Don't complain about the length of your son's hair if you're asking him to assume significant family responsibilities that you can't handle. If your daughter finds relaxation in loud music, recognize that your back problems may also be causing stress and tension for her. Decide what things are really important to your health and to the happiness of your family, prioritize them, and satisfy them whenever possible. Don't waste time worrying about the incidental things.

Maintaining joyful family relationships through a prolonged disability requires a lot of hard work. If you ignore your family and dwell only on your own needs, you may develop an unhappy family life that may be difficult to change.

16. SOCIAL LIFE

Most people enjoy the companionship of others in social situations. Going to movies, plays, sporting events, church activities, school functions, or dinner parties brings happiness and builds strong friendships. Unfortunately, bad-back problems can cause a person's social life to vitually disappear.

This chapter describes some of the factors that may affect the social lives of people with bad backs. It also provides suggestions for staying socially active in spite of recurring back problems.

SOCIAL DILEMMAS

It is difficult for a host or hostess to invite someone in pain to an event that's supposed to be fun. The pain of the one who is suffering may detract from the enjoyment of other guests or from the spontaneity of the event. If the host or hostess is more concerned with staging the activity than with the happiness of the guests, a person in pain will probably not be invited. But if the host or hostess seeks to serve the pleasure of the guests, additional steps will be taken to accommodate special needs of someone who has a bad back.

People with bad backs may attempt to maintain social activities as though nothing was wrong. Extra doses of painkilling drugs may be taken in unsuccessful attempts to mask intense pain and discomfort. But it is usually quite obvious to a host, hostess, or social companion when a bad-back victim is either in pain or under the influence of medications. Offers to help the person in pain are often rejected as unneeded. An attempt to be stoic and hide what is obvious to others can easily create an unpleasant social situation.

People with back pain may discover previous social companions to be consistently unavailable. Bowling teams and golf partners may seek healthy replacements for those who can no longer participate. Healthy people don't generally dislike those who are sick or disabled. They just don't want their social activities restricted by someone who is disabled.

A husband or wife may frequently have to attend social events alone if one spouse is bedridden with back pain. After a while, the healthy spouse—like one who is divorced or widowed—may choose to avoid or ask not to be invited to social events that are planned primarily for couples. This often places healthy spouses in double-bind situations. They may feel an obligation—or sincere desire—to attend a social function, but at the same time, they feel guilty about leaving their bedridden mate at home. On the other hand, they may not want to go in the first place, but they attend in order to fulfill a perceived social obligation. Subsequent dissatisfaction on the part of either spouse could lead to marital stress and tension.

The demands of children can also be troublesome. Standing in below-zero weather to watch a hockey game, or sitting on an uncomfortable chair through an entire piano recital can be very painful. If an event comes at the end of a particularly stressful day, a parent with back problems may not be physically capable of attending. Unless the child understands and accepts the social limitations of the parent, nonattendance can create disappointment and hard feelings.

SOCIAL GUIDELINES

If you want an active social life, there are several steps you can take to ensure it. Here are some basic guidelines you can follow.

Inform Your Friends. Let those close to you know what your limitations are. If you find it difficult to stay seated in one position for any length of time, say so. Be straightforward and honest about your physical limitations. Make it clear that you would like to continue to be socially active with your friends, but to do so will require some adjustments. Let your friends know that cutting back on your social activities is no reflection on them. Tell them also that you hope they remain friends during this difficult period.

Consult Your Diary. You should be keeping a diary. Consult it frequently to confirm your limitations. Maybe your back condition prevents you from standing or sitting for extended periods. Maybe certain days of the week, or times of the day, are particularly bad if you follow routine activities. Document the activities that cause pain in your back, and keep track of the things that make you feel good. Use your diary to plan enjoyable, pain-free social activities.

Establish Priorities. You are obviously limited by your bad back, so the number of events in which you can participate should be selected with care. You may find, for example, that dinner parties and children's concerts cause equal amounts of discomfort and pain. You should neither give up the parties nor the concerts in favor of one over the other. Plan instead to set aside time for both. Explain to your friends the need to attend your children's performances, and explain to your children the need to get out and be with your friends. You should convey to both the fact that your condition is temporary, and as soon as you can overcome your bad back, you'll be able to attend everything that time will allow.

Tell It Like It Is. Many people have difficulty in handling the social pressures of drinking. They tend to yield when offered additional drinks. This is suicidal for someone with a bad back who is taking a combination of muscle relaxants and painkillers. Make it clear to those with whom you socialize that you cannot mix medication and alcohol. If you need help in refusing, say so.

If you must excuse yourself from a sitdown dinner to rest on a bed or couch, do it. But tell your host or hostess ahead of time that you may need a place to lie down if your pain gets out of hand. Be concerned about disrupting the party, but don't push yourself beyond your limits. If you're having muscle spasms, you will cause more disruption by displaying your agony.

Develop Alternatives. If your back problems prevent you from continuing the vigorous activities you once enjoyed, develop alternative pastimes. A family swim makes a good outing and provides beneficial hydrotherapy. Picnics with short hikes allow you to sit in the sun and relax and get needed exercise in walking. Card games, scrabble, or backgammon may serve as substitutes for plays, movies, or concerts if you can play while stretched out on a sofa or couch.

If you like to entertain, but can't handle the work involved, get your friends together for potluck dinners. Change your style of entertaining to conform with your temporary limitations and pain.

The recreation and companionship found in an active social life can provide valuable therapy for overcoming your bad back. Like other forms of therapy, however, you must aggressively work to maintain an optimum level of involvement. A passive response to social limitations may lead to loneliness and depression.

17. DOCTORS

The complexity of your back problems makes your choice of a doctor extremely important. It's not easy, however, to find the doctor who is best suited for you and your problems. Several different doctors specialize in back problems, but the treatments they employ are not unique to their field of specialization. Different approaches may be used by doctors practicing the same specialty, or the same approach may be used by different specialists.

This chapter discusses general doctor-patient relationships, identifies specialists who deal with back problems, and provides suggestions for dealing with all doctors, regardless of their field of specialization.

DOCTOR-PATIENT RELATIONSHIPS

Most doctors are very busy. Their time is extremely valuable and in short supply. Back problems, however, take time to resolve. Recognizing this, some doctors will reserve extra time for their bad-back patients. Other doctors will treat the bad back as an acute condition, prescribing pills, heat treatments, rest, or braces for a short-term recovery. But if a doctor diagnoses a chronic back condition as being acute, healing will be very difficult.

Psychological factors, such as stress, anxiety, frustration, and depression, are involved in back disorders as often as physiological problems. The cause of bad backs is often elusive, and when found, it is sometimes difficult to treat.

Not all doctors are experts on bad backs, nor should they be expected to be. But the ego of some doctors prevents them from admitting a professional inadequacy. It is extremely unfortunate for a person with a bad back to encounter a doctor who doesn't know what is wrong or what can be done to help, and who will not confess a lack of knowledge. In that case, the patient's self-direction is all that's available for coping with pain and discomfort.

Even more serious is the situation in which the doctor knows what can be done, does not have the expertise to do it, and will not refer the patient to another doctor who can help. And in other cases, doctors may prescribe an inadequate or incorrect remedy because they don't know the right one, or they know the right one but don't know how to do it, and they feel the patient wouldn't know the difference.

A doctor who specializes in back disorders will know and understand the dynamics of the patient's problems. Valuable time will be judiciously spent in recognition of the long-term nature of the ailment. All possible treatments will be openly discussed, regardless of the specialists who perform them. Every reasonable alternative will be evaluated, and the patient will be encouraged to seek additional information and consultation. The potential long-term dependence on drugs or apparatus will be acknowledged, and a program of careful drug usage will be prescribed.

Many people can't tell if they have the wrong doctor. Continued back problems should serve as a clue or as an impetus for seeking help elsewhere. Once a skilled bad-back practitioner is found, relief should occur rather quickly. Back pain doesn't have to be a lifelong ailment. A good doctor will ensure that it isn't.

SPECIALISTS

There are at least seven specialists who include back problems in their professional practice. The difference in their training and procedures is as varied as the professional regard they have for each other. The degree of expertise about bad backs that each possesses is not necessarily a factor of their specialty, their place of training, or the facility in which they practice. Each has a different theory about why backs hurt and what can be done about it.

Brief descriptions are provided here in alphabetical order for the specialties of acupuncture, chiropractic, internal medicine, neurology and neurosurgery, orthopedics and orthopedic surgery, and osteopathy. The descriptions should not be considered inclusive. Individuals within each specialty may concentrate on total treatment of bad backs or on only one aspect of the ailment. On the other hand, a specialist may focus on everything but the back and know only the rudiments of back problems.

Acupuncture. This form of surgical procedure was devised in China many centuries before Christ. The practice of acupuncture involves insertion of needles of various metals, shapes, and sizes into one or more of 365 specific locations on the torso, arms, legs, and head of the patient. Acupuncture is supposed to relieve internal congestion and restore equilibrium to bodily functions. It has been used to treat a wide variety of diseases, including arthritis, headache, convulsions, lethargy, and colic. Acupuncture is also used to treat chronic back pain.

In theory, the insertion of needles into the body stimulates small nerve fibers to send impulses to the brain where they register as acute pain. When the signals are received in the brain stem, they trigger counterimpulses that travel down the spinal cord and close off chronic pain impulses.

Acupuncture has been effective in stopping muscle spasms and in relieving various types of back pain. It would not, however, be used to correct a herniated disc that was pressing on spinal nerves.

Chiropractic. This medical specialty is based on the premise that all bodily systems and physiological functions are controlled by the nervous system. Interference with control of these bodily systems impairs their operation and induces disease by rendering the body less resistant to infection and other agitating causes. Chiropractic includes the manipulation of various structures of the body, especially the spinal column, to relieve disorders that are thought to be abnormal functions of the nervous system. Chiropractic manipulation is also used to restore normal motion or nerve function that has been impaired by a partial dislocation or sprain.

Many people have found chiropractic to be very helpful in correcting their back problems. If treatment is carried out early in the history of the ailment, surgery may be avoided. In cases where surgery is required, however, deliberate manipulation may seriously aggrevate existing problems.

Internal Medicine. This branch of medical practice deals with the treatment of organic illnesses that do not require or are not amenable to surgical treatment. Internists are highly qualified in the art of diagnosis and nonsurgical treatments. If their diagnosis suggests surgery, they will refer their patients to appropriate surgical specialists.

A person with a bad back will probably see an internist before any of the other specialists. This is very appropriate, since back pain can come from one of several sources, including kidney disorders, infections, or tumors. The internist, being a skilled diagnostician, might discover problems that could be overlooked by other specialists.

Neurology and Neurosurgery. Neurology is concerned with the structure and function of the nerves and the nervous system. It deals with diseases of the brain, spinal cord, nerves, and with organic disturbances of nerve cells.

Neurosurgery is the branch of medicine that deals with the surgical treatment of nerve tissues. The neurosurgeon operates on injuries, diseased conditions, and congenital defects of the brain, spinal cord, peripheral and autonomic nervous systems, and of the structures that cover them.

Since back pain usually comes from abused nerve tissues, a neurosurgeon or neurologist may quite likely be the specialists to whom a back patient will be referred. In performing back surgery, a neurosurgeon generally is most concerned with correcting damage to nerve tissue and in alleviating pain. Although neurosurgeons perform the same operations as other surgeons, their approach reflects their area of specialization.

Orthopedics and Orthopedic Surgery. Orthopedics involves the correction or cure of deformities and diseases of the spine, bones, joints, muscles, or other parts of the skeletal system.

Orthopedic surgery is the branch of medicine that is devoted to the surgical prevention, correction, or alleviation of deformities, especially of the spine, arms, and legs. Orthopedic surgery is distinguished from general surgery by the extensive use of mechanical appliances, including corsets, braces, and plaster casts. Orthopedic surgeons, whose main focus is on damaged bones, joints, and muscles, perform many back operations. A patient will often be referred to an orthopedic surgeon when it is thought that the structures of the back are damaged or diseased.

Osteopathy. This specialty is based on the doctrine that all diseases are due to abnormalities in or near joints, and that the treatment of every disease involves correction of these abnormalities. The osteopath treats these abnormalities by manipulations, which are designed to restore the musculoskeletal system to its normal state. If no precipitating disease is apparent, manipulation alone may be used, anticipating that relief will be obtained in a large percentage of cases. If pain and discomfort continue, rest, physical support, mechanical traction, heat, diathermy, exercise, and muscle-relaxing drugs are used according to the nature of each individual case.

Osteopaths use manipulation as an adjunct to, not as a substitute for, accepted methods of treatment. This is especially true if recognized disease states are present.

It's important for you to know that the way you deal with your doctor will probably have as much impact on your recovery as the specialization that is involved.

DEALING WITH DOCTORS

Lawyers say a man who chooses to defend himself has a fool for an attorney. The same could be said for people who choose to treat their back problems without the aid of a doctor. Probably no other ailment has so many old wives' tales and misconceptions associated with it. Some people are afraid that every doctor wants to operate on their bad back, and if they have surgery, they will be crippled for life. Nothing could be further from the truth. There are good and bad doctors just as there are good and bad lawyers, bankers, auto repairmen, politicians, and clergymen. If you deal with a doctor in a professional way, you will generally get professional treatment. If you're not open and honest with your doctor, you have only yourself to blame for continued problems. But if your doctor is obviously mistreating you, make an appointment to see someone else.

Here are some suggestions for dealing with doctors, regardless of their area of specialization.

Study Your Condition. Read as much as you can about your back problems, and try to discover why they exist. This book contains some basic informaton, but there are several other sources you should consider. The bibliography at the end of this book contains a lot of material that can be found in your public library. Read as much as you can, and don't pass lightly over the technical terms. They will probably be used when you discuss your problems with your doctor.

Study diagrams of bodily areas that are involved. Draw pictures of your back after looking at illustrations in books. That will help familiarize you with the functions and interrelationships of all parts of your back. Learn as much as you can about your entire body, because you will find areas other than your back are usually involved in back problems in one way or another.

It has already been suggested that you maintain a diary, keeping track of social activities, weight, medications, emotions, and the outside weather conditions. Detailed information about your condition will assist your doctor in planning your treatment program.

Ask Questions. Your doctor's time is very valuable. To conserve time and still get the most for your money, ask brief but specific questions about your condition, not about what you heard happened to someone else.

If your doctor puts you off, is vague, or obviously does not know the answers to your questions, start looking for another doctor. Do so even though the one you're now seeing may have been recommended by a relative, close friend, or your employer. Remember that overcoming your back problems is more important than protecting the sensitive feelings of your doctor or friends.

Good doctors will give you good answers, or tell you where you can find them. Don't forget they want you to get well too. If you're unhappy or still in pain, your doctor will also be unhappy. Ask your questions and stay with your doctor until you get the answers you're looking for. If your doctor is unfamiliar with certain aspects of your problem, ask for other sources, such as a book or another specialist. Offer to share with your doctor the information you discover. The two of you working together should be able to resolve your back problem sooner than either one of you working alone.

Here are some of the questions you might want to ask your doctor.

1. What are the potential side effects of the medications you are now prescribing for me?
2. What kind of exercises can I safely do?
3. What would cause my back to get worse? better?
4. What will the treatment cost? How long will it take?
5. What specifically do you expect of me if I am to follow your prescribed treatment? What things should I not do?
6. What are some other types of treatments? Why is yours better? Where can I find about other methods?
7. How successful have you been in treating bad backs? Can you give me names of patients that I can contact?

Make a list of these and other questions that continue to bother you. Leave a copy with your doctor in case more time is needed to provide the answers.

Hang On To Your X-rays. Your X-rays belong to you. You paid for them and are entitled to them. Take them home so you can compare them with what you have been reading, or with what your doctor has told you. Learn how your back is put together and how to identify where problems exist. If your radiologist won't explain your X-rays to you, ask your doctor to go over them to point out any problems that might exist.

You will never be able to read an X-ray like a specialist. But if the problems are pointed out to you, and you've done your homework, you should at least have a better understanding of your problems. Later, if back surgery is contemplated, you will have a better base of information on which to make your decision.

Your X-rays should be kept at your radiologist's or your doctor's office for future reference, so be sure to return them when you feel you have studied them long enough. You can get them back at a later date if necessary.

If you want your X-rays sent to another doctor, you can have them mailed. Your radiologist, or whoever has the X-rays, may charge you for postage, but they should not hesitate to send them to other specialists. This is very important, especially if you are seeking another opinion. It will save the expense of having additional X-rays taken.

Seek Other Opinions. You have the right to seek another opinion regarding your condition. A good doctor will welcome verification of a diagnosis along with additional information you may obtain. Only an unprofessional doctor will complain, so use that as a cue for seeking out another doctor.

When dealing with your doctor remember that it's your body that hurts. If your doctor says nothing else can be done for you, ask what alternatives were pursued in arriving at that conclusion. If you feel certain that other approaches exist, seek them out, and inform your doctor accordingly.

A doctor's main concern should be with you, your pain and agony, and your pressing desire to get well. Your primary physician should not get upset if you ask that your records be sent to another specialist. If resistance is expressed, consider another primary doctor, or demand to know why another opinion is not acceptable. Be aware of some of the nonmedical aspects of referral. They are often politically motivated and sometimes have social overtones.

At the same time, don't jump on every healing bandwagon. If a referral has introduced you to a new or radical method for correcting back problems, check it out thoroughly. Ask the practitioner for evidence of successful treatments. Talk to other patients who have been treated by the method. Talk to your primary doctor about the procedure. If you decide to undergo the treatment, be sure you clearly understand all of the potential consequences.

When seeking other opinions, remember the differences between specialists. At the center of your problem lie bones, muscles, nerves, and cartilaginous discs. An orthopedic surgeon specializes in the bones and joints. A neurosurgeon concentrates on the nervous system. They both may perform the same general type of back operation, so choosing between them may be very difficult. Your eventual choice will unquestionably affect the outcome of your back condition. This holds true for other specialists as well.

Establish An Overall Treatment Program. You and your doctor should develop an overall treatment program that includes diet, exercise, drugs, and work and leisure activities. Establish a time schedule for each part of your program, but don't set a specific date on which you expect to be free of pain. If you're not painfree on the appointed date, the psychological feelings of failure could mask actual improvements that are apparent in the accomplishment of individual program segments. Your hoped-for outcome is freedom from pain, but your primary focus should be placed on reaching single goals within the total program.

Set realistic goals that can be met. Goals that are difficult to reach may prove psychologically frustrating. Goals that are too easy to accomplish may produce no beneficial effects.

There are several goals worth pursuing. You could establish a plan for losing weight or for beginning and progressing through an exercise program. You could also establish a schedule for reducing your drug intake. If you can achieve these and other goals, you should be well on your way toward overcoming your bad back.

It is important to include your doctor in your treatment program so your progress can be medically evaluated. Diets, exercise, and drug management should not be attempted without your doctor's advice, suggestions, and encouragement.

You need to trust and have faith in your doctor, or your recovery will be long and difficult. Compassion, empathy, and a sincere desire to make you well are as important as your doctor's area of specialization. If the cause of your problem is not addressed directly, you may be left to depend on medications and your own devices. A good doctor, on the other hand, should be able to guide you to a rapid and lasting recovery from your bad back.

18. DRUGS AND ALCOHOL

Because of the nature of bad-back problems, many people tend to seek their relief from drugs and alcohol, even though the combination of the two substances can be extremely dangerous. Unfortunately, those who are seeking an escape from pain, don't always know what they are consuming or what effect it is having on their bodily functions.

This chapter discusses some of the problems that can be caused by the use and misuse of drugs and alcohol. It also presents a number of suggestions for avoiding drug- or alcohol-related problems in the treatment of bad backs.

BACK PROBLEMS AND DRUGS

Many people who suffer from chronic back pain are dependent—physiologically or psychologically—on one or more drugs. This happens because many doctors find it easier to prescribe drugs than to try to understand and eliminate the underlying causes of pain.

The two major groups of drugs that are prescribed for people with bad backs are tranquilizers and painkillers, both of which are discussed here.

Tranquilizers. These drugs are prescribed to reduce stress and tension that can trigger painful muscle spasms. In 1977, 60 million prescriptions were written for the tranquilizer Valium (diazepam), making it America's most widely prescribed drug. Librium (chloriazepoxide hydrochloride), a chemical relative of Valium but considered to be about one-fourth as potent by weight, is the third most prescribed drug. Other well-known tranquilizers include Equanil and Miltown (both meprobamate).

According to separate studies reported by the *New York Times* and the National Commission on Marijauna and Drug Abuse, approximately one out of six Americans takes some form of tranquilizer regularly. Statistics also reveal that tranquilizers are taken by 72 percent more women than men.

Tranquilizers are right behind alcohol, nicotine, and aspirin as the Nation's most abused drugs. There are far more prescription-tranquilizer users in the United States than there are illicit drug users.

There is no firm evidence of a death resulting from an overdose of Valium but the drug can blunt reflexes if overused. This makes such activities as driving extremely dangerous. Accidental death may result, but it is not due directly to the use of Valium.

Contrary to popular belief, Valium poses few problems for moderate social drinkers. The drug does, however, increase the level of intoxication. If Valium is taken in combination with moderate quantities of alcohol, problems similar to those accompanying gross intoxication can occur.

Alcohol and tranquilizers are both central nervous system depressants. They slow down such important functions as thinking, reasoning, and breathing. They also slow the heartbeat and reduce the power of the senses. Therefore, if large quantities of alcohol and tranquilizers are consumed together, bodily functions will be slowed down to the point of stopping. And if they stop, death will occur.

On the positive side, Valium is very effective in breaking muscle spasm and pain cycles that are so devastating for bad-back sufferers. The tranquilizing effect of Valium reduces stress and tension and allows a person in pain to move about freely.

The real danger with tranquilizers lies in the fact that they are so widely and freely prescribed and so readily available. This is unfortunate, because much of the muscle tension and anxiety that accompanies a bad back can be relieved by nonpharmaceutical approaches, such as massage and exercise. Many forms of physical therapy can produce the same calm, relaxed states that are experienced with tranquilizers.

Painkillers. Analgesic drugs and drug compounds, such as Demerol (meperidine hydrochloride), Percodan, Empirim, and Darvon, are prescribed to reduce or eliminate pain. Although pain pills often bring blessed relief for the person with a bad back, their continued use can delay treatment of underlying causes. Pain serves to notify a person that something is wrong with bodily functions. Reliance on pain pills without attacking the cause of the pain can actually prolong a person's agony. The patient and the doctor should both recognize that in a majority of cases, pain is only a temporary condition that will hopefully be gone before the initial prescription is used up. Instead of masking pain, painkillers should be used diagnostically to discover the source of the patient's problems.

DRUG-RELATED PROBLEMS

Adverse reactions indicate that some drugs are inherently toxic. Most cases of toxicity, however, are direct consequences of intentional or inadvertent drug misuse. A common type of misuse involves the consumption of two or more drugs at the same time, allowing them to act simultaneously within the body.

The term *synergism* is used to characterize any interaction that produces a combined drug effect greater than the sum of the effects of the individual drugs. The opposite of synergism is *antagonism*. In the context of drug misuse, an antagonistic effect is produced whenever the desired action of one drug is diminished or completely eliminated by the biological action of another drug.

The extent to which drugs interact synergistically or antagonistically is dependent upon the degree of control each has on the other's absorption, distribution, excretion, or biotransformation. Absorption refers to the incorporation of drugs into the bloodstream. Distribution refers to the movement of a drug from the bloodstream to the part of the body where the drug is to take effect. Excretion refers to the manner by which a drug is discharged from the body. Biotransformation refers to the manner in which a drug affects the chemical and physical changes of organisms and cells that are necessary for maintaining life.

For example, if barbituates (sedatives) and alcohol are taken together, the combination can cause a person to stop breathing, even though the individual dosage would not be expected to kill if the two substances were taken separately. The adverse synergistic effects stemming from consumption of barbituates and alcohol can be attributed to the competition between the two drugs for the same system of enzymes that are responsible for their biotransformation. These enzymes do not have the capacity to simultaneously metabolize both drugs at rates equal to the individual metabolic rates. Thus, if a person takes prescribed sleeping pills soon after leaving a cocktail party at which alcoholic beverages were consumed in moderation, the competitive interaction between alcohol and barbituates for metabolizing enzymes will result in the retardation of both alcohol and barbituate biotransformation. The net effect would be an enhanced central nervous system depression, possibly equivalent to that resulting from the consumption of a lethal barbituate overdose. In short, the combination could be deadly.

The key to avoiding drug-related problems is to know how to handle narcotic substances, either individually or in combinations.

HANDLING DRUGS AND ALCOHOL

If you're a social drinker and are now taking pain pills and tranquilizers, you would be wise not to mix the drugs and alcohol. Admittedly, that's easier said than done. There will be, or have been, times when your back pain is almost unbearable. At the end of a day of pill taking and continued pain, a couple of stiff drinks may be very appealing. The pain may not disappear, but the alcohol may wash away your concern over it.

You should recognize two obvious dangers when combining drugs and alcohol. First, if you stay home and become intoxicated on drugs and alcohol, you could seriously injure yourself. Statistics of the National Safety Council verify that most serious accidents occur in the home. If your condition caused you to fall or stumble, you could aggrevate your bad back, or disable some other part of your body.

Second, if you were foolish enough to leave home while intoxicated, you could end up injuring yourself and someone else. A personal injury lawsuit on top of your existing medical expenses could result in serious financial hardship for you and your family.

There are a number of specific things you can do to avoid the problems that can be caused by drugs and alcohol. Several of them are presented here.

Learn About Drugs and Alcohol. You should find out everything you can about drugs and alcohol and the effects they can have on you, especially when they are taken together. Your local library and your doctor are both good sources of information. So are pharmaceutical companies, since they must document the effects and hazards of the drugs they produce.

Understand Your Prescription. Ask your doctor why certain drugs are being prescribed and what role they have in your overall treatment program. Know how the drugs are supposed to affect your bad back. If you are concerned about side effects, ask if there are alternative drugs that are just as beneficial. If your doctor can't answer your questions, talk to your local pharmacist.

Keep track of your drug intake. For each type of pill, write down—in your diary—the time of day and the way you were feeling when you took it. See if there are times when you are taking pills only to follow a prescription, and not because you need them. Ask your doctor or your pharmacist if you can take your pills only as needed. You may be able to cut down your drug intake considerably. Some drugs must, however, be taken periodically to be effective. Find out which type of prescription you have been given.

If drug taking has become a habit instead of a response to an obvious need, you may be heading for trouble.

Understand Your Needs. Know and understand what your bodily conditions are that require medication. Ask your doctor if pain pills or tranquilizers have been prescribed to keep you comfortable, or to prevent recurring muscle spasms and other conditions. Objectively determine your tolerance for pain, stress, and tension, and relate the use of drugs to your specific circumstances. Don't use drugs if your body doesn't need them to get better.

Establish Reasonable Deadlines. Since you are not going to stay on drugs forever, find out from your doctor when you will be able to get along without them. The deadline can either be a calendar date, or a time when your body has reached a specific point of recovery. Emphasize to your doctor that you want to eliminate the cause of your pain as soon as possible. Don't forget that back problems generally take a long time to correct, but time spent using drugs may be wasted if the cause of your bad back is not being treated directly.

Limit Your Alcohol. You don't have to completely abstain from drinking, but you are asking for trouble if you drink too much. Aside from causing all sorts of complications in combination with drugs, consuming too much alcohol can cause you to gain weight. The added weight can add stress to your back and subvert a well-intentioned exercise program.

Set aside specific times—preferably with dinner—when you can have a drink or two. Determine how much alcohol you should have and stick with whatever limits you set. You should also consider wine instead of distilled spirits; it's much better for you and less inclined to add extra pounds.

Avoid Combinations. Don't mix pills and alcohol regardless of the situation. If you've been invited to a cocktail party, you may have to decide between pills, which you may need to get through the night, and alcohol, which you may enjoy much more. The best choice would be to take the pills and forsake the alcohol. You may still hurt the next day, but you'll feel psychologically better for having gone to the party, and you won't have a drug and alcohol hangover. If your social companions won't accept your excuse for not drinking, you might be moving in the wrong social circle.

Seek Alternatives. Instead of having a drink or taking a tranquilizer at the end of the day, pamper yourself with a hot shower. If you have access to a health club, use the whirlpool bath for 15 or 20 minutes before you go to bed. If a health club is unavailable, see if a nearby motel has a whirlpool that you can use or rent until you get better.

Instead of taking a pain pill so you can sit at your desk for an extra hour, get up and go for a short walk. The exercise will do you good, and so will the psychological break in your work.

Switch from drinking hard liquor, which has no nutritional value, to wine, which is much better for you. Wine drinking can be enjoyable as well as educational. You can even make wine at home. It's fun, and it may serve as a good substitute for more vigorous hobbies.

Avoid stress- and tension-producing events that cause you to rely on tranquilizers. Actively seek alternative ways of relaxing. Discover the things that cause you to have pain, and substitute accordingly.

The key to avoiding drug-related problems is to know how to handle narcotic substances, either individually or in combinations. You must also eliminate your dependence on drugs and alcohol and use them carefully and judiciously. If you keep your head clear and approach your back problems head-on, your recovery will come a lot sooner.

19. STANDING, LIFTING, SITTING, AND SLEEPING

Studies involving thousands of bad-back sufferers have reported that four out of five backaches were caused by the accumulated effects of poor posture, improper lifting of heavy objects, and bad sleeping conditions. Serious back disorders were caused by spontaneous bursts of activity that could not be supported by weakened muscles.

This chapter explains some of the problems associated with standing, lifting, sitting, and sleeping. It also contains suggestions for properly engaging in these essential activities.

STANDING

People have often been urged to adopt a military posture: chest out, shoulders back, and pelvis forward. This is a very unnatural position that can cause serious problems for a weak back. The forward curve of the spine in the lower back is accentuated, leading to swayback or lordosis. This excess curvature places stress on the rear edge of the intervertebral discs, especially those in the lumbar region. If the discs are already weakened, the stress can cause herniation and sciatic pain.

Sometimes, swayback comes naturally. As people get older, their stomach muscles weaken and a potbelly develops. Their spines, in the lower region of the back, bend forward slowly but sharply, leading to swayback. As the stomach starts to sag, the chest begins to droop, and the shoulders drop. All of this shifting puts the back out of balance. Physiological functions are disturbed, and muscles and ligaments are thrust into an abnormal state of tension and strain.

Swayback is the most significant problem associated with the way people stand. But it is also found in other activities like lifting, sitting, and sleeping.

LIFTING

Lifting can cause more problems for the back than any other activity. In 1970, two Swedish researchers found that lifting the wrong way—with legs straight and back bent at the waist—imposed pressures of more than 500 pounds per square inch on the L3 disc. Proper lifting by comparison imposed a load of only 227 pounds per square inch, or about half the stress. Normal standing imposes pressure of 182 pounds per square inch so the effects of lifting can be quite substantial, especially if lifting is done incorrectly.

It was also found that back stress generally is affected more by the size and shape of an object being lifted than its weight. A small 35-pound object held close to the body adds about 250 pounds of force to the vertebrae of the lower back. If the 35-pound object is enclosed in a large box and held farther from the body, pressure on the lumbar vertebrae is increased to about 900 pounds per square inch.

Pushing is a lot like lifting, because it involves many of the same muscles. And it can be just as painful if done incorrectly or in excess. Pushing a vacuum cleaner or grocery cart can cause tremendous pain no matter how careful you are. That's because the muscles in your lower back, hips, and buttocks are all involved.

Most people bend their back slightly to overcome the force of inertia needed to get the objects moving. Using vacuum cleaners and grocery carts involves a lot of starting, stopping, and changing directions, so the back muscles are called on repeatedly. That's like bending slightly to lift an object over and over again. Even though the distance is not great, the force required to overcome inertia may be, especially if the objects are heavy.

If you continue to bend over after the object is moving, your lower back muscles will continue to work to keep you from falling over. Once inertia is overcome, there is no counterbalancing force to keep you upright. It's no wonder that a person with back problems experiences pain after grocery shopping or vacuuming.

SITTING

Sitting is generally more difficult than standing because your body is no longer supported by your legs. Body weight is centered instead on your lower back and hips.

A lot of folklore exists about the kinds of chairs that are good and bad for people with back problems. Soft, overstuffed chairs should be avoided, but the alternative should not be a hard, straight-backed chair as many people believe. Support of the back and comfort should be the major concerns.

The seat of a chair should provide a comfortable cushion. If chronic back pain is present, a soft seat is needed to soothe aching muscles in the buttocks and hips. These muscles cannot relax and be comfortable if the seat is as hard as slate. In addition, your body weight needs to be cushioned and absorbed. If your discs are weak, they may be unable to absorb all of the pressure that's placed upon them. The soft seat will carry part of the load, whereas a hard seat will just transmit the stress back to your spine.

Support for your lower back must also be provided. A straight-backed chair may force you into an unnatural position that is difficult to maintain for any length of time. The back of your chair should fit the natural contours of your spine with added support provided for the stress-laden lumbar region. Secretarial and most contour chairs provide excellent support.

If armrests are used, it's easier for the muscles of the shoulders and upper back to hold your torso upright. Your arms can contribute to the support of your back when they come in contact with the armrests.

SLEEPING

Sleep is supposed to be a period of rest, during which the powers of the body are restored. But rest and comfort will only come if sleeping is done properly.

The spine is most comfortable when it assumes its natural curves. If your body lies in a position that is in opposition to normal curves, muscles and ligaments will work continuously to correct the position. If you awake in the morning with a sore back, it's probably because your muscles and ligaments are exhausted from working all night trying to return your back to its normal position.

Most of your body weight is in your hips and shoulders. Accordingly, these two areas need the greatest amount of support when sleeping. But most mattresses are built uniformly, with equal support given to all parts of your body. An ideal mattress is one that will accommodate your shoulders and hips, but will also keep the middle of your back in its normal position. If your mattress is really good, you could lie on either side and your spine would be in a straight line.

A board placed between a mattress and an innerspring will not help a bad back. If your mattress is too soft, you will still sink in, down to the rigid board. Efforts to modify a poor mattress with a board or other means is a waste of time and money. If you have back problems you would be much better off investing in a good mattress rather than trying to improve a poor one.

HELP YOUR BACK

You will help your back considerably if you develop good habits for standing, lifting, sitting, and sleeping. Here are some suggestions for preventing future problems and alleviating damage that has already been done.

Stand Tall. A quick test will indicate how good your posture is. Stand with your heels, buttocks, shoulders, and head against a wall. If there is space between the wall and your lower back, you have too much arch or swayback. Shuffle your feet forward so your back slides down the wall. Rotate your pelvis backward and tighten your abdominal muscles. Slide back up the wall into the starting position. The space between your lower back and the wall should be much smaller. The purpose of this test is to demonstrate how much you should flatten out the spinal curves in your neck and lower back.

To stand and walk tall, tilt your pelvis backward, throw your chest up and out, and pull in your abdominal muscles. Keep your chin down, and don't allow your stomach to sag or your hips and pelvis to tilt forward. Keep a shallow curve in your lower spine so excess pressure will not be placed on your lumbar vertebrae. By standing

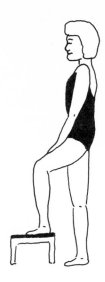

FIGURE 8. STANDING WITH ONE FOOT ELEVATED

tall, the stresses of standing and walking will be uniformly distributed all along your spinal column, and you will not subject weak areas to excessive stress.

You can also reduce muscle tension and swayback by elevating one leg while standing as in figure 8. Like most people, you probably arch your back a little to keep your balance. Raising your foot to a rail or stool will flatten the arch and help you stand erect.

The worst way to stand is to lean forward with your hips and pelvis against a sink, counter, or table top. This forces you to hold your shoulders back to maintain your balance. It also deepens the curve in your lower back and causes swayback. If you have to lean forward, use a footrest or bend your knees so you can reduce muscle tension and pressure on the discs in your lower back.

Men and women should both avoid using high heel shoes if they have back problems. The heels cause you to bend the top half of your body backwards to maintain balance. This causes swayback as well as unsteadiness.

For some reason, most bathroom sinks at home and in motels are built at waist level or lower. This makes it very difficult for men to shave when their backs hurt. An average-size man must bend down repeatedly to wet his face or rinse his razor. If you have this problem, shave with your knees bent or shave at the kitchen sink, which is usually much higher. This will eliminate swayback and reduce pressure on the lumbar discs.

Lift Properly. Remember that your lower back acts as a hinge or fulcrum when you lift. It was made that way, and normal lifting shouldn't cause problems. But when degenerated discs cause weakness in the hinge, back problems will generally occur if lifting is done improperly.

In lifting any object, be sure to get as close to it as possible by moving either yourself or the object. Bend your knees so you're squating down next to it, and keep your back bent slightly. Grasp the object with both hands so you're sure you have a feel for its weight and shape, and then lift by standing up, as shown in figure 9. This action uses the large muscles in your thighs instead of the smaller

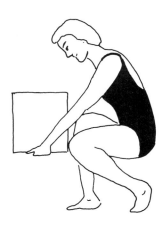

FIGURE 9. CORRECT METHOD OF LIFTING

muscles in your back. Keep the object close to you as you straighten up, and don't twist or turn your body. Continue to keep the object close to your body as you carry it and set it down, because carrying and placing objects can be just as stressful as lifting.

You should use your arm and leg muscles in addition to your back muscles when lifting. If you rely only on your back muscles, they may suffer additional injury if they are already sore and tender from muscle spasms. You should also avoid using your back muscles to push or pull, since that can be just as painful as lifting.

Never try to lift a heavy object alone. Always get someone to help you. And before you start to lift, think about what you are going to be doing. Decide who is going to lift what part of the object. Don't make quick movements that will place added stress on your muscles, and don't lift anything over your head. Holding an object directly above you makes your back sway and centers additional stress straight down your spine where it's absorbed by the lumbar discs.

If you have a lot of back pain, you should get into the habit of not lifting or pushing at all. If you encounter a friend, neighbor, or

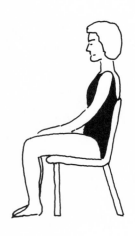

FIGURE 10. SITTING STRAIGHT

stranger whose car is stuck in a snowbank, don't be foolish enough to offer to push. If you feel compelled to help, offer to drive for assistance. When traveling, don't carry your luggage to avoid paying a tip. The current rates for tipping are a lot less than the cost of missed work or additional visits to your doctor's office that could result from straining your back muscles.

Try to get someone else to do your grocery shopping and vacuuming. In short, you should avoid any movements that add stress and strain to already sore and tired muscles.

Sit Straight. When you find a comfortable chair, be aware of how you sit in it. Be sure to keep the lower part of your back against the supporting area that is provided. Avoid swayback, because it will place too much stress on the discs in your lower back. Figure 10 illustates the correct way to sit.

The worst thing you can do when sitting is to slump down in the seat. Your weight would then be supported by the back of your neck and your pelvis. It's much better to sit up straight so your weight is evenly distributed up and down your spine.

Remember, while you are sitting, the muscles in your back are still working to support you and keep you upright. Because they are working, they will get tired if they are not allowed to rest. That's why you should not sit for extended periods of time, particularly in one position. You should get up and walk around occasionally to shift the weight of your body to your leg muscles, giving your back muscles a well-deserved rest. Crossing your legs while sitting will also relieve some of the stress on your back.

You can reduce physical stress on your spine and on the ligaments and muscles that support it if you keep one or both of your knees higher than your hips when sitting. This is best accomplished with a small stool; not with a very low chair, because difficulty in getting in and out of a low chair will neutralize the effects of having your knees raised. If a stool is unavailable, at least be sure that both feet are touching the floor and that your knees are not lower than your hips.

The way you sit in and drive an automobile can have a significant impact on your back problems. Bucket seats, like those found in sports cars, provide much better support for the lower back than do seats in standard sedans. If you keep your seat too far back while driving, you will have to stretch your legs forward to reach the pedals, producing harmful swayback. For the most comfortable ride, move your seat forward so you don't have to stretch your legs. A back cushion for your car seat can be used if it supports the lumbar region of your back. If it creates an improper curve in your back, don't use it.

Sleep Comfortably. The key to getting a good night's sleep is to find a comfortable position that provides support for your back. Probably the best position is to lie on one side with your head supported by a pillow and your knees slightly bent. In this position, your hips and shoulders will be slightly recessed into the mattress and your spine will be in a horizontal line.

The second best position would be to lie on your back with your head on a moderately firm pillow. Another pillow inserted under your knees will lower your pelvis and leave your spine bent in a natural position. If you keep your legs straight while lying on your back, you will develop some swayback, since your pelvis will be extended upward.

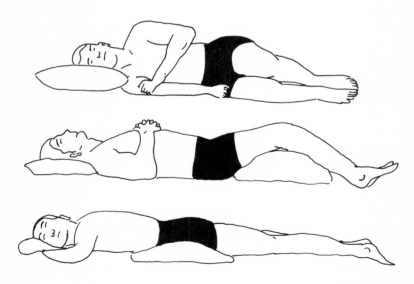

FIGURE 11. SLEEPING POSITIONS

Sleeping flat on your stomach is the worst thing you can do. It causes swayback and strains the muscles of your shoulders and back. It may, however, be difficult for you to switch to another position if you've slept on your stomach all your life. If you feel you must sleep on your stomach, place a pillow under your hips. That will raise your buttocks and take the sway out of your back. The three sleeping positions are shown in figure 11.

Getting in and out of bed is as important as the position in which you sleep, especially if you have to get up a lot during the night, or if you lie down frequently during the day. In either case, you should avoid making quick movements that can place unnatural stress and strain on tired and sore muscles, resulting in muscle spasms.

The first thing to do in getting out of bed is to turn on your side, close to the edge of the bed. One arm should be beneath you and the other should be resting on top of your body. Place the hand of the top arm palm-down near your face. Push your hand against the bed to raise your body, and at the same time, drop your legs over the edge of the bed to the floor. This will cause you to pivot into a sitting position. Pull your feet close to the edge of the bed so they are right under you. Bend forward slightly to balance yourself, and then use your hands and thigh muscles to raise yourself to a standing position. Figure 12 shows the correct way for getting out of bed.

Getting into bed is equally important. Lower yourself slowly to a sitting position at the edge of the bed. Let your leg muscles do most of the work in getting you there. Using your hips as a pivot, lower your head and side to the bed, and at the same time, swing your legs up on to the bed. You should find yourself lying on your side with your knees slightly bent. This is a good position to stay in, but if you want to move, do it slowly and carefully so you don't put extra stress on your back muscles.

It's always a good idea to get your blankets and pillows positioned before you lie down so you avoid getting up and down more than necessary.

If you take care of yourself and work at it, your bad-back condition should only be temporary. If it looks as though you are in for a long seige, however, you may want to rent a hospital bed or modify the bed you have. You can bring your bed to hospital height by having someone raise it on cement blocks.

If you need a new mattress, be sure to shop carefully. You spend about one-third of your life in bed, so investing in a good quality mattress is well worth the price you have to pay. You might also consider buying a water bed. Many people with back problems think they're great. They offer excellent support and the heaters they have help to soothe tired and sore muscles.

Concentrate on how you stand, lift, sit, and sleep. Make deliberate movements, and avoid unnecessary stress and strain. If you are careful in the way you do these things, you will shorten the time needed to overcome your bad back.

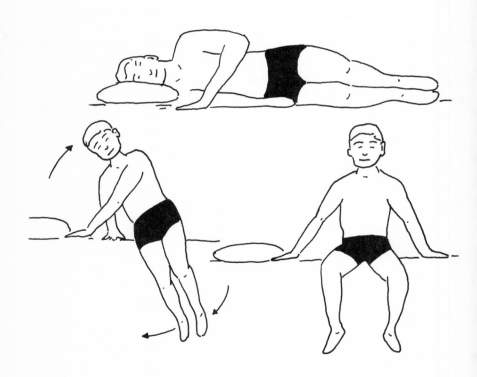

FIGURE 12. GETTING OUT OF BED

20. DEPRESSION AND POSITIVE ATTITUDES

The psychological aspects of pain and disability are every bit as important as the physiological aspects. If you are depressed, hold negative attitudes, or are under emotional stress, your healing process will be slowed dramatically. It's important to understand how psychological forces can affect your back problems, and it's equally important to know what can be done to counter those forces and speed your recovery.

This chapter deals with the effect that psychological depression has on back problems. It also discusses the role of positive attitudes in overcoming a bad back and offers suggestions for maintaining healthy attitudes toward yourself and others.

DYNAMICS OF DEPRESSION

Depression is a neurotic condition, characterized by dejection and despair, in which people take a defeatist or hopeless attitude toward the things that bother them. Depression is a normal, short-term response to an unhappy external situation, such as a death in the family, severe financial problems, or chronic illness. Depression, dejection, and despair are frequent companions to prolonged back problems and pain. If depression becomes a long-term condition, additional symptoms may develop, and serious mental problems may result.

Unconscious hostility is the central dynamic factor in many depressive reactions. Typically, people who are in poor health will direct their hostility toward family members or others with whom they come in close contact. People with bad backs tend to blame their condition on doctors they feel are incompetent, employers they think expect too much, children they feel can't do anything for themselves, and spouses they feel lack understanding and empathy. This unconscious hostility usually causes guilt feelings when the bad-back victim recognizes that other people are not at fault. Subsequently, guilt causes hostility to be turned inward, resulting in feelings of unworthiness, self-depreciation, and despondency. A vicious cycle begins that's difficult to arrest.

Depressed people often don't know how to act when things are going well. They fail to recognize even the slightest improvement in their condition and focus instead on how much pain and discomfort still remains. When others recognize and acknowledge improvement, depressed people respond with more hostility, feeling that their pain and suffering is being ignored. Guilt again follows hostility, and depression continues.

An important change in the human psyche is in operation between the ages of 35 and 45. Statistics show that both men and women are more acutely aware of approaching age, and for some, that can become unbearable. When the age crisis is compounded by a debilitating back problem, the probability that a depressive reaction will occur is greatly increased.

Statistics also show a rise in the frequency of mental depression in men who are about 40 years old. This is the age when back problems also tend to occur. When compared with men, women generally experience depressive reactions at an earlier age, although back problems tend to occur at about the same time.

Because of the indeterminate nature of depression, effective treatments are not easy to prescribe. In spite of this, the prognosis for depression is usually quite good. In the majority of cases, depression disappears as the person's condition improves or is otherwise altered. For many people, maintaining a positive outlook on life has been a very effective way of dealing with depression and its affiliated problems.

POSITIVE ATTITUDES

Your attitudes toward your back problems will have a significant effect on how rapidly you recover. The frustration of day-to-day pain and the inability to do the things you want can make you feel very depressed. A positive attitude, although essential for your mental health, is extremely difficult to maintain if you hurt all the time.

Many self-help books are available for developing and maintaining positive attitudes. Reading them may give you the psychological lift needed to get through your most difficult days. Some of the books are written by people who have had unhappy experiences of their own. They found keys to happier living that could possibly be applied to your life. Read their books and you may obtain valuable information for preventing or overcoming depression.

Your ability to maintain a positive outlook on life hinges on your attitudes toward others and yourself. If these attitudes are negative, there is no way you can sustain a healthy disposition.

ATTITUDES TOWARD OTHERS

The worst thing you can do for your mental health is to become hostile and bitter, especially toward other people. That's because the scars of hostility can last a long time. To avoid such hostility, you should take several things into consideration.

First of all, it is very difficult—if not impossible—for anyone, including your doctor, to understand how a bad back feels or what problems it creates unless he or she has had similar experiences. And with each bad-back condition a wide variation exists in the amount of pain and disability that is present. So people who say they know how you feel may know exactly or have no idea at all.

Secondly, other people will be concerned about the way you feel, and they will ask about your condition because they want to know. Recognize the sincerity of their concerns, but don't belabor the issue by going into extensive detail. Other people will be as frustrated as you are with your continued back problems, and they may be very disappointed with what you tell them. They will not be angry with you, only with the fact that you continue to hurt.

Finally, your pain will not disappear suddenly as if by magic. But after it is gone, you will find it difficult to pinpoint the day you really began to feel good. Others around you will sense that you are in less pain. If they recognize your improvement, give them the benefit of their perceptions and thank them for their concern. Don't be angry with them if they fail to acknowledge that you still hurt.

You may be so wrapped up with your pain that you won't know if you're better or not.

ATTITUDES TOWARD YOURSELF

The attitudes you hold toward yourself are also very important. You may agonize over the fact that you do not seem to be getting better no matter what you do. You can become discouraged, embittered, angry, and hard to live with. It takes a great deal of effort to stay happy when you hurt, and yet, you must if you don't want your spouse to leave you, your children to turn against you, your employer to fire you, or your friends to desert you. Here are some definite steps you can take to help you maintain a healthy attitude.

First, accept the fact that you have a bad back for whatever reason. Second, if you are experiencing a lot of pain, accept the fact that it will probably stay around for quite a while, at least a lot longer than you would like. Third, accept the fact that even when you think you have your back problem under control, it may come back again to haunt you.

Keep a diary and lay out a plan of attack. Periodically assess your condition and make changes when necessary. If you are overweight, set a goal to lose extra pounds and carry out your diet with a vengence. Since you won't be able to burn off calories with vigorous exercise, you are going to have to reduce your intake and not eat or drink as much as you have.

Assess your drinking habits, especially if you rely on alcohol to ease your pain and misery. Drinking adds calories and it can play havoc with your body if you're taking any medication. Consider wine as a substitute for hard liquor. It tastes good, complements a diet, and is better for you.

A new wave of energy will come over you and give you a happier outlook on life if you can break one bad habit or develop a healthy habit and stick with it. If you can ward off depression and develop a positive attitude toward life, you will be well on your way toward eliminating your bad-back problems.

21. SUMMARY OF PART II

Back problems involve much more than bones, discs, muscles, and nerves. For many people, back pain and disability have brought on an entirely new life style. No other ailment can have such a devastating impact on as many aspects of daily life. Some people have been told, or led to believe, that they must capitulate to their back problems and learn to live with them. Nothing could be farther from the truth.

Part II presents a multitude of suggestions, which allow people to aggresively overcome problems they are experiencing in several critical areas. It tells what should be done at the onset of back problems, and it prescribes ways of dealing with back problems that last for long periods. It suggests several specific courses of action that can be very helpful in a wide variety of situations.

Part II also deals with stresses of the work environment, and it offers suggestions for coping with employment problems that are precipitated by bad backs. It discusses some of the problems that people encounter when they try to modify their sexual activity to accommodate continued back problems. It discusses the stress that families experience when one member has a bad back. It also discusses family reactions to that stress, and provides suggestions for coping with problems that occur. It describes some of the factors that can affect the social lives of people with bad backs, and it provides some suggestions for staying socially active in spite of recurring back problems.

Part II also discusses general doctor-patient relationships, and provides suggestions for dealing with all doctors, regardless of their field of specialization. It discusses some of the problems that can

*be caused by the use and misuse of drugs and alcohol, and it presents
a number of suggestions for avoiding those problems. It also describes some of the back-related problems associated with standing,
lifting, sitting, and sleeping, and it offers suggestions for properly
engaging in those essential activities.*

*Finally, Part II deals with the combined effect of psychological
depression and back problems. It also discusses the role of positive
attitudes in overcoming a bad back, and offers suggestions for
maintaining healthy attitudes.*

*Part III deals with the ways in which bad backs are diagnosed
and treated.*

PART III

DIAGNOSIS AND

TREATMENT

22. KNOWING WHAT TO DO AND DOING IT

Diagnosis is the key to effective treatment, because no cure can accurately be prescribed for any condition until the cause is clearly understood. If a diagnosis is incorrect, recovery could be due to chance, regardless of how effective the treatment may be. If a diagnosis is correct, and the treatment poor, chance may again guide the recovery. Between the two, diagnosis and treatment, the greater possibility for recovery lies with a correct diagnosis.

Diagnosis can be carried out in several ways, from a physical examination to the use of sophisticated electrical and chemical systems. In the end, however, a diagnosis is only as good as the person making it.

Treatment of back problems can vary greatly among practitioners. Some doctors prefer conservative treatments—bed rest, heat, massage, and exercise—and shy away from surgery of any kind. Other doctors see specialized surgery, when done properly, as a godsend for a person with chronic back pain.

Treatment of the psyche is often called for, especially if back problems are serious and long-lasting. These treatments can also vary, from extensive psychotherapy to simple methods of relaxation.

Part III deals with some of the more common diagnostic techniques and methods of treating bad backs. You're the one who will have to decide which procedure best serves your needs. You will be able to make your decision with the help of a qualified professional, experience of other bad-back victims, and material you get from books like this. The material contained in Part III should assist you in knowing what to do and how to go about doing it.

23. DIAGNOSIS

The initial diagnosis of your back problems will probably be done by an internist, who may also be your family doctor. An internist is probably the best person to start with because of the enigmatic nature of back problems. Your back pain could be the result of disease or injury to one or more of your internal organs. The pain could also come from disruption of the internal processes of your body. If the internal organs are involved, your internist is the one practitioner who can do the most to help. But if your back problem involves muscles, ligaments, bones, or discs, you may be referred to an orthopedic surgeon, neurosurgeon, or some other specialist.

This chapter discusses a variety of procedures for diagnosing back problems, including physical examinations, assessment of pain, and the use of sophisticated chemical and electrical instrumentation.

PHYSICAL EXAMINATION

The first thing your doctor will do in the physical examination is document your medical history. You can help by recalling events that may have led to the problems you are now experiencing. Injuries, illnesses, or family disposition to back problems, should all be documented. Your doctor will decide what is and what is not important, so provide as much information as you can.

Prepare yourself for your examination by making a list of all your past illnesses and injuries, especially those that caused you back pain. This will save valuable time and help your doctor focus on your immediate problems.

116

Your doctor will also want to know if you are experiencing problems or pains when coughing, sneezing, or going to the bathroom. The location and description of pain will also be checked. Your doctor will want to know if your pain feels like throbbing, burning, pins and needles, or if all you can feel is numbness. You should also tell your doctor if your pain is located only in your back, or if it travels into your legs, ankles, feet, and toes.

You will be asked to stand and move about so your doctor can see if you are favoring one position, or if pain registers on your face as you change positions. Your doctor will also look to see if you list to one side or if you have a pronounced swayback. Throughout the examination, you may be asked to stand, sit, lie down, or bend over to touch your toes. Your doctor will even observe your breathing while you talk to see if it is painful or difficult.

Your doctor may administer a number of tests that will be directed toward specific disturbances in your back. These tests have been developed over the years by specialists who have worked with thousands of people like you who have had back problems. Many of the tests are named after the practitioners who developed them.

The tests are relatively simple, but the results can be very useful in diagnosing back problems. In one test, you will be asked to lie on your back and raise one leg. You should be able to raise it 80 to 90 degrees. Your doctor, while holding your leg and working against your efforts, will ask you to bend your toes or your foot backwards and forwards. You may also be asked to turn your ankles in or out, again acting against the pressure of your doctor's grasp.

Some of the tests can be very painful for a person with a bad back, but pain is one of the things your doctor will be looking for. It will help pinpoint the location and type of problems you've been experiencing. It's not an attempt to hurt you, only to learn more about your bad back. Be aware of this and explain as best you can where and how you hurt. Trying to hide your pain will only confuse the examination. And unless your doctor gets all the facts about your bad back, a precise diagnosis may be difficult to make.

Some of the tests measure sensitivity of your nerves. Your doctor will place a sharp needle or a dull instrument against your body, and you—without looking—will have to describe the sensations you feel. Again, it's very important for you to give accurate information. But because of your back pain, you may have to concentrate very hard to give the correct response.

During the tests, you may be asked to stand erect, lie on your back, lie on your stomach, or sit in a chair. In each instance, you will be asked to move particular parts of your body, usually in opposition to the grasp of your doctor. The tests may prove difficult, but they all have a purpose, so do everything that is asked of you.

If you've been given a complete examination, and if you've been able to provide useful information, you should know what your problems are after one visit. To compile additional information, however, your doctor may ask you to submit to laboratory tests, X-rays, or further examination by specialists. If your doctor says something else is needed to make the initial diagnosis complete, don't hesitate because of costs. You may end up paying a lot more if you don't get a complete diagnosis in the early stages of your back problems.

PAIN

The type of pain you are experiencing will tell a lot about the nature and location of your back problems. If your pain throbs or pulsates at a fairly constant nuisance level until a motion of some sort causes intense pain, you probably have a severe, low-back muscle strain. Your condition probably does not involve a damaged disc.

If your pain travels down one or both of your legs and into your buttocks, feet, toes, and ankles, a herniated disc or other substance is probably pressing on one or more of your peripheral nerves.

If you experience pain when you awake in the morning, but find the pain decreasing as the day progresses and your body movement increases, it may be arthritic pain. This type pain may recur when you get tired or are overly active. You may also hurt because of poor sleeping conditions. If your muscles have to work all night to get you into the right sleeping position, they will be sore and tired when morning comes. A poor mattress that fails to support your muscles can also be a source of morning pain.

Record your pain experiences in your diary. Over time, your record will help your doctor in continued diagnosis and treatment of your back problems.

X-RAY

A widely used diagnostic technique that you will probably encounter is X-ray. An X-ray examination can reveal two major back problems. The first is vertebral displacement in which the vertebrae do not line up properly because one or more have moved forward or out of place. Vertebral displacement or dislocation can result from an injury or a congenital defect in the structure of the back. In either case, improperly aligned vertebrae may not be able to provide the support needed for normal bodily functions. Pain will occur when the displaced bones press on adjoining nerves.

X-rays can also reveal the distance between two intervertebral discs, although the results of such findings may be confounding. If the space between two vertebrae has narrowed, it may indicate a disc has herniated or collapsed. On the other hand, a narrow disc space does not necessarily signify a collapsed disc. It may only reflect a smaller than normal disc. And even if the disc has collapsed, it may not be causing pain unless it is pressing on a nerve. If pain is experienced, it may be totally unrelated to the apparent compressed disc space.

The nonbony parts of the back—ligaments, tendons, muscles, and discs—show up poorly on X-rays. But these nonbony parts are often the major culprits in back pain. Because of this and other factors, diagnosis of back pain should not rest on the basis of one set of X-rays. Additional tests are generally needed to obtain a complete diagnosis.

MYELOGRAM

Sometimes a myelogram is needed to confirm an earlier diagnosis and locate the level of a herniated disc. A myelogram is an X-ray photograph that is taken after a radiopaque substance has been injected into the spinal canal. The production of myelograms is called myelography.

In preparation for the myelogram, you will be strapped, face down with your back exposed, to an X-ray table that can be tilted into a number of different positions. Your doctor will insert a needle into your spinal canal and will draw out between 6 and 12 cubic centimeters of a watery liquid called cerebrospinal fluid. With the needle still in place, your doctor will replace the cerebrospinal fluid with a radiopaque substance containing iodized poppy-seed oil. This substance will show up as a sharp contrast on X-ray film.

The radiopaque substance is generally injected into the L2-L3 disc space, and there are a number of reasons for this. About 80 percent of all disc problems occur at the L5-S1 level. Another 19 percent occur at the L4-L5 level. Inserting the substance above those areas will ensure adequate coverage when the table is tilted. It will also prevent additional pain by avoiding those areas of your back that already hurt. Tender nerves could suffer additional trauma if the needle was inserted directly into an area where trouble was suspected.

The table on which you will be lying will be tilted so the radiopaque substance can travel up and down the spinal canal. You could be placed upright in a vertical position, upside down, or anywhere in between.

While you are being moved, an X-ray image of your back will appear on a fluoroscope screen above the table. Your doctor will watch this screen to observe movement of the radiopaque substance as the table is moved into different positions. If a tumor or herniated disc is bulging out into the spinal canal, an indentation should appear in the darkened image of the radiopaque substance. Your doctor will take an X-ray picture at that spot before you are moved to another position.

While the myelogram is being administered, the cerebrospinal fluid that was taken out will be subjected to laboratory tests to check the protein level. A slight rise above normal levels would indicate spinal irritations. A large increase in protein is indicative of a possible tumor or spinal infection. The results of these tests will be given to your doctor as soon as possible.

After X-rays are taken, your doctor will withdraw the radiopaque substance from your spinal canal, a band-aid will be placed over the point where the needle was inserted, and you will be asked to rest for a period of 12 to 24 hours. Some people feel nauseous after a myelogram; others have bad headaches. The discomfort could be attributed to the fact that the body works hard to replace the cerebrospinal fluid that is taken out for testing. The reactions to myelography usually vary from individual to individual, however.

If a ruptured disc has herniated into the spinal canal, the myelogram should show it. In about 15 to 25 percent of the cases, however, the myelogram either fails to show the herniation, or it gives false information. Herniation is most frequently missed when a ruptured disc does not protrude into the spinal canal. A disc can bulge off to one side where it can still press on one of the peripheral nerves. In that case, pain symptoms may be more useful than the myelogram.

If a question remains about a possible disc herniation, your doctor may prescribe a discogram.

DISCOGRAM

A discogram is an excellent diagnostic test for disc herniation. Discography follows much the same procedure as myelography except that the radiopaque substance—a water soluble dye—is introduced directly into the nucleus pulposus of a suspected disc. The procedure is also different from a myelogram in that you lie on your side on an X-ray table that remains stationary during the test. Generally, novocain is injected into the disc ahead of the dye to reduce pain and discomfort.

Like myelography, an image of your vertebrae is projected on a fluoroscope screen above you. When the dye is injected into a disc, your doctor will be taking X-ray pictures of any abnormalities that appear. If a disc has herniated, it should show up clearly on the screen.

Discography is a painful procedure compared to myelography, but the pain is an aid to diagnosis and lasts only a matter of minutes in most cases. Essentially, the injection of dye into the disc will cause a re-enactment of the type of pain you experienced in disc herniation. This brief episode of pain enables your doctor to investigate and interpret your back condition at its worst.

Because of the pain and discomfort, a discogram is generally not administered unless your doctor wishes to confirm a diagnosis made prior to or in contemplation of back surgery.

A discogram is 100 percent accurate in revealing pathological changes in the discs. The discogram will also reveal a normal disc with an intact annulus fibrosis and a normal nucleus pulposes. But if the annulus fibrosis has ruptured or degenerated, the discogram will show the exact location of the rupture, regardless of where it occurs in the disc. The discogram will also indicate whether the rupture is confined to the intervertebral disc or if it has extended into the spinal canal.

In spite of the fact that it is sometimes painful, a discogram is probably the best diagnostic procedure for suspected disc problems. Other tests, such as an electromyogram, can be used for less serious cases.

ELECTROMYOGRAM

Electromyography is another test used in the diagnosis of back problems. During this test, the electrical potential generated by muscle fibers is amplified, and the signals are recorded on tape or played through a loudspeaker. An experienced electromyographer can distinguish many abnormalities simply by listening to the sounds that are produced.

Electromyography requires insertion of very fine, coated needles into various muscles in the back, legs, or arms, depending on where pain is felt. The solid needles have wires in their centers, allowing them to pick up electrical impulses from very localized areas of muscle fiber.

If a nerve supplying a muscle has been destroyed, the muscle becomes so irritable that electrical potentials are generated almost all the time, even when the muscle is relaxed. Electromyography, in recognizing these electrical potentials, often makes it possible to locate irritative or destructive lesions by testing various muscles in the body. Knowing which nerves innervate which muscles, your doctor can study abnormal electrical potential in specific muscles and discover, for example, that a herniated disc is pressing on a specific nerve root.

In certain cases, conduction velocity studies are done. By stimulating a nerve at one point, and then picking up the electrical wave as it passes another point, or as it produces a muscle contraction, a doctor can determine the speed at which messages travel in the nerve. Pressure on nerve roots can disturb conduction, and primary nerve disease may alter the speed of conduction.

A good diagnosis will not only clarify your symptoms, it will also identify the cause of your problems. The next step will then be to establish and carry out an appropriate treatment program.

24. EXERCISE

Studies have shown that as many as 80 percent of all bad backs are due to poor muscle tone and lack of exercise. Regardless of the severity of your problem, length of time you have had a bad back, or number of surgeries you have had to endure, you can find some improvement and possibly a cure through exercise. Many doctors feel the only way to overcome a bad back is through a program of therapeutic exercise applied to specific problem areas and muscles.

This chapter describes some of the benefits that exercise can provide as well as some of the dangers that should be avoided. It also suggests several specific exercises that can be very helpful in overcoming back problems.

BENEFITS OF EXERCISE

Many people loathe exercise. They feel it takes too much time, is an inconvenience, and causes perspiration and body odor. They would rather consume pain pills and muscle relaxants than do even the simplest exercises. Yet, exercise done regularly can do more for a person with a bad back than hundreds of pills.

A great deal is known about the effect of exercise; how it strengthens muscles, increases blood flow, improves respiration, assists in weight loss, and saves money over medications. In contrast, many questions remain about the side effects of some of the drugs that are prescribed for bad backs. Common sense indicates that for most conditions, it is better to exercise than to take pills.

Exercise has tremendous benefits in terms of cost and convenience.

Thousands of dollars in medical and hospital costs can be avoided by engaging in daily forms of exercise. Exercise can also save time that would otherwise be spent in doctors' offices, in hospitals, or flat on your back in bed.

If someone offered you $10,000 in cash to start a moderate program of exercise, you would quite likely accept the offer. The $10,000 is probably what it would cost you in initial medical bills if you didn't exercise and allowed your back problems to get worse through deterioration of back and stomach muscles. Brief periods of exercise once or twice a day could very well be the best—and least expensive—medicine you can find. It's almost like putting money in the bank.

You should not have to be coaxed into exercising if you really want to overcome your bad back. Exercise has guaranteed and proven results. The misery you experience with your back problems must surely be greater than the perceived inconvenience of starting an exercise program.

If you can improve the tone and strength of the muscles of your back, sides, stomach, and chest, you will significantly reduce stress and pressure on your intervertebral discs. A program of regular exercise, started early after the onset of back problems, can probably eliminate the need for surgery and extensive hospitalization. If you have already had back surgery, a planned program of exercise can hasten recovery.

A WORD OF CAUTION

Don't start your exercise program until you check with your doctor, because you can cause further damage to your back by doing the wrong exercises. Your doctor can recommend the specific type, number, and frequency of exercises that are best for you.

Swimming, bicycling, and walking are excellent forms of exercise. They do not involve abrupt movements, and they tend to strengthen abdominal muscles. Activities that involve jarring or unpredictable movement, such as jogging, tennis, and skiing, can cause additional problems for your back.

Even with the best exercises you have to be careful. If you choose swimming, you should avoid sudden and significant changes in temperature between the air and the water that might trigger muscle spasms. If the water is cool, take a shower before you swim to gradually lower your body temperature. If you are not careful, you can lose all the benefits of exercising by provoking your muscles into spasms.

YOUR EXERCISE PROGRAM

Exercising does not have to be vigorous to be beneficial. The calesthenics you did when you were younger—push-ups, sit-ups, leg raises—were for young and flexible muscles. They may not be appropriate now. The exercises that affect the muscles in the stomach and back are often subtle, but always effective.

Start with the exercises doctors have found to be best. Then after the pain is gone, your stomach firm and flat, and you've lost some weight, you can start doing the more vigorous calesthenics you hated to do when you were younger.

Begin your exercise program carefully and slowly. Don't be alarmed if the exercises cause some mild discomfort that lasts a few minutes. If the pain is significant and lasts more than 15 or 20 minutes, stop! Don't do any more exercising until you have seen or talked to your doctor.

You should do your exercises on a firm surface covered with a thin mat or heavy blanket. Always start your exercises slowly and in a prescribed order to allow muscles to loosen up gradually. You can help tight muscles relax before you start exercising by applying heat or massage.

The first goal of back exercises is to relax and stretch the muscles that support the spinal column. The second goal is to strengthen all of the muscles that support the spinal system, with special emphasis on the abdominal muscles. These two goals are achieved with an exercise program that emphasizes slow and deliberate movements and has frequent periods for rest or relaxation.

There are several exercises for stretching and strengthening your muscles. Eight of the most common ones are presented here. At first glance, they don't appear as though they would do much to help. Remember, however, that your back and stomach muscles have been under stress and strain for quite a while. They are probably quite tender and unable to work through strenuous exercises. The last thing you would want to do would be to injure them by making them work too hard.

The first four exercises listed here help to stretch and loosen your muscles. The second four help to strengthen them. For maximum benefit, the exercises should be completed in the order in which they are presented. Try to do as many repetitions of each exercise as your back muscles will allow. Push for improvement, but don't bring on additional trauma. Most important of all, keep your doctor informed of your progress.

Lateral Trunk Stretch. This exercise will loosen and stretch the muscles on either side of your torso. Lie on your back with your knees bent and your hands behind your head. Cross your right leg over your left just above the knee. Press down on your right leg and straighten out your left leg until the inside of your left knee touches the floor. Hold for a count of five and then return your legs to the starting position. Next, cross your left leg over your right leg. Press down again until the inside of your right knee touches the floor. Count to five, and then return to the starting position. The press with both legs constitutes one repetition. You should start with five repetitions. See figure 13.

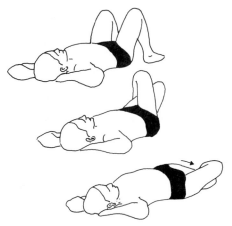

FIGURE 13. LATERAL TRUNK STRETCH

Pelvic Tilt. This exercise will stretch and loosen your gluteus maximus muscles—your buttocks. Lie on your back with your knees bent, your feet on the floor, your head on a small pillow, and your hands behind your head. Tighten the muscles in your stomach and buttocks at the same time so your lower back is pressed flat against the floor. Hold for a count of five, which is one repetition. Do five repetitions. A modification of this exercise can be done while you are standing with your back pressed against a wall. See figure 14.

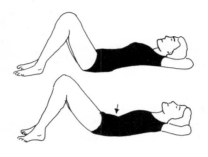

FIGURE 14. PELVIC TILT

Knee to Chest Raise. This exercise will stretch stiff and tightened muscles, ligaments, and joints in the lower back. Lie on your back with a small pillow under your head, your arms at your sides, your feet flat on the floor, and your knees bent. Raise one knee and clasp it to your chest with both arms as tight as you can without causing pain. Count to five, keeping your shoulders flat on the floor. Release your knee and slowly lower your leg to the starting position. Clasp your other knee to your chest, again count to five, and release. Finally, clasp both knees to your chest and hold for a count of five. Release and slowly lower both legs to the starting position. These three movements constitute one repetition. Start with five, and gradually work your way up to ten repetitions. See figure 15.

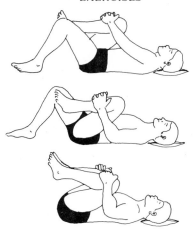

FIGURE 15. KNEE TO CHEST RAISE

Single Straight-Leg Raise.This exercise stretches and loosens the hamstring, buttocks, and hip muscles. Lie on your back with your feet on the floor, your knees bent, and your hands behind your head. Straighten your left leg, and with your knee rigid, raise it as high as you can until you develop pain or tightness in your thigh. Hold for a count of five. Slowly lower your leg until it is flat on the floor. Return your left leg to the starting position with the knee bent, then straighten your right leg and do the same exercise. Working both legs constitutes one repetition. Do five repetitions. See figure 16.

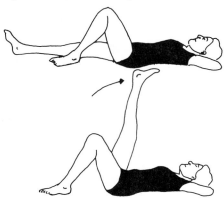

FIGURE 16. SINGLE STRAIGHT-LEG RAISE

Half Sit-Up. This exercise will strengthen the muscles of your abdomen and lower back. Lie on your back with your knees bent and your hands across your chest. Raise up and touch your hands to your knees without raising your lower back from the floor. Hold yourself in this position for a count of five. Return to the starting position for one repetition. Do five repetitions. See figure 17.

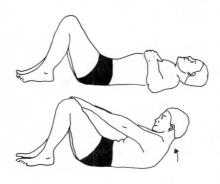

FIGURE 17. HALF SIT UP

Nose To Knee Touch. This exercise strengthens your abdominal muscles and stretches your hip muscles. Lie on your back with your feet on the floor and your knees bent. Pull your left knee up and clasp it to your chest while simultaneously extending your right leg as far as you can with the knee rigid. Keeping your lower back against the floor, raise your head and touch your left knee with your nose. Hold in that position for a count of five. Slowly lower your head to the starting position, but continue to grasp your knee to your chest. Rest a moment, then raise your head and touch your nose to your left knee again. Do this nose-knee touch five times. Then lower your left leg and return to the starting position. Rest again, then bring the right knee up to your chest and repeat the exercise for one repetition. Do five repetitions. See figure 18.

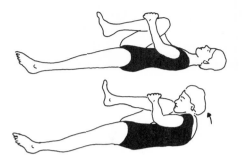

FIGURE 18. NOSE TO KNEE TOUCH

Scissors. This exercise will stretch out and strengthen your hamstring, lower back, and hip muscles. It will also strengthen your stomach muscles. Lie on your back with your feet on the floor, your knees bent, and your hands behind your head. Bring your knees up to your chest, and then straighten your legs out above you. Slowly scissors your legs back and forth 10 times in a walking motion. Then criss-cross them 10 times, left over right, right over left. Return your knees to your chest, then slowly lower them to the starting position for one repetition. Do five repetitions. See figure 19.

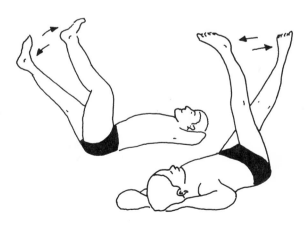

FIGURE 19. SCISSORS

Hip Hyperextension. This exercise stretches and strengthens your hip muscles, buttocks, and lower back muscles. Lie on your stomach with your arms extended out in front of you. Stiffen your left leg, and make the knee rigid. Raise the leg from your hip, keeping your pelvis flat on the floor. Lower your leg and then raise it again a total of five times for one repetition. Rest, then straighten your right leg and repeat the exercise for one repetition. Do five repetitions with each leg. See figure 20.

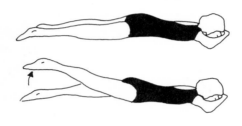

FIGURE 20. HIP HYPERTENSION

There are many exercises you can use to strengthen your abdominal and back muscles. Once you feel comfortable with basic movements like those described here, move on to more strenuous exercises, but only after you have talked with your doctor. As your muscles become stronger, you will be able to develop an exercise routine that will provide long-term relief from your back problems.

You should be aware, however, that not all bad-back conditions can be corrected by exercise. Surgery may possibly be a much more appropriate treatment.

25.BACK SURGERY

Surgery involves the treatment of diseases, injuries, or deformities by manual operation and manipulation or by using instruments and appliances. Many people think of surgery in terms of anesthesia and cutting. It is that, but it is also much more.

This chapter describes the nature of back surgery and three of the most common surgical techniques that are now being used to correct back problems.

CONSIDERATION OF BACK SURGERY

Although surgery can be dramatic, it often is the best possible treatment for certain back problems. Some acute conditions, such as fractured vertebrae (broken back) or massive rupture of a disc, require emergency surgery. Sciatica and spondylolythesis are frequent causes of prompt spinal surgery. Infections, tumors, and arthritic conditions are less frequent, but often urgent reasons for surgery.

Statistics reveal that about 5 percent of all people with some type of back problem have corrective surgery.

Most people are very cautious about surgery. They prefer to explore more "conservative" forms of treatment such as rest, exercise, and heat therapy. In many cases, those treatments provide lasting benefits. On the other hand, delaying necessary surgery may prolong the healing process and bring on additional problems.

There are two major kinds of back operations: laminectomies and fusions. A laminectomy is performed to remove material— usually a herniated disc—that is pressing on spinal nerves. A fusion is done to stabilize the back by locking adjoining vertebrae together so there is no motion between them. Variations in the two procedures are developed by specialists who apply their unique skills and knowledge to the surgical relief of back disorders.

A third operation, chemonucleolysis, involves the injection of a chemical substance into the disc space where it dissolves the degenerated nucleus pulposes.

The basic elements of all three procedures are discussed in the paragraphs that follow.

LAMINECTOMY

The surgical procedure for removing herniated disc material is called a laminectomy. It involves partial or total removal of the laminae, which are thin plates of bone that form the back part of the spinal canal.

A laminectomy begins with a horizontal or vertical incision about four inches long in the middle of the back. The incision is made over the spinous processes; the bony ridges you can feel when you rub your hand up and down the middle of your back. The surgeon cuts through the skin, the huge strap muscles that lie on each side of the vertebrae, and the posterior ligaments that run down the back of the spine. This incision exposes the posterior surfaces of the bony vertebrae. The surgeon will carefully chisel or saw an opening about the size of a dime in the lamina on either side of the spinous process. The covering over the spinal canal is then cut to expose the spinal cord.

Using a bright surgical spotlight, the surgeon looks through the opening made through skin, muscle, ligament, and bone, and carefully studies the material that's pressing on the spinal nerves. The myelogram or discogram taken a day or two before surgery will be used to accurately guide the next moves of the surgeon. With extreme gentleness, the spinal nerves will be moved aside to expose the herniation. The surgeon may notice an indentation in the spinal cord, resulting from the pressure of the protruding disc.

In most cases, the herniation is a white, pea-sized piece of disc that is fibrous and stringy, much like crab meat. Using a long instrument, the surgeon will snip out that part of the disc that is imposing pressure on the nerve roots. If the vertebrae are subsequently to be fused, the entire disc will be taken out. The portion that is removed will not be replaced.

Occasionally, the material pressing on a nerve root is not from a herniated disc. It could be fragments of bone, created by a vertebral fracture. Bone spurs, deposits from arthritis, or scar tissue could also press on the nerve roots.

The laminae play only a small role in the supporting function of the vertebrae. Partial or total removal of one or two laminae does not significantly interfere with support or motion of the spine. This is not always true for the discs, however.

In removing part or all of a disc, the surgeon is also removing some of the cushion from between two vertebrae. If the remaining portion of the disc continues to degenerate, the cushioning effect may be completely eliminated, and a subsequent fusion will have to be performed to stabilize the spine and prevent the vertebrae from rubbing together.

The success rate for laminectomies ranges from 30 to 80 percent, and is dependent upon a number of variables. The skill of the surgeon who performs the operation, the hospital in which it is performed, and post-operative care all play important parts in a patient's recovery. Another important factor is the way the patient behaves after having surgery.

FUSION

The back operation designed to stabilize vertebrae, or to stop motion between them, is called a fusion. It involves the fusing (biological gluing) of bones into a solid mass. Fusion is almost always used to correct slipped vertebrae and vertebrae that have been attacked by tuberculosis or arthritis.

Spinal fusion is done by many surgeons in combination with a laminectomy to correct a herniated disc. The dual procedure tends to stabilize the spine by preserving the space created when disc material was removed between two or more vertebrae. The most successful type of spinal fusion is one in which the entire disc is removed and replaced by several bone plugs or pieces of bone.

The operation begins with either a vertical or horizontal incision in the skin directly over the affected area. The muscles and the posterior ligaments are cut and pulled back to expose the vertebrae. After making the initial incision, the surgeon may pursue one of several procedures, all of which contain similar elements.

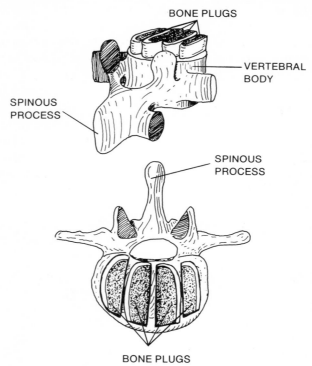

FIGURE 21. POSITION OF BONE PLUGS IN FUSION

The vertebrae are cut at selected sites with a chisel and mallet, layer by layer, until bleeding of the bone occurs. Then bone is taken from another part of the body or from a bone bank and wedged, wired, or otherwise fastened to the freshly cut vertebrae. The procedure actually consists of a bone graft or a bone transplant.

Figure 21 illustrates one example of bone placement for a fusion. The intervertebral disc has been removed and replaced by four bone plugs.

Once bone is sawed or chiseled away from its blood supply, it will die. Later, when it is wedged tightly against raw, living bone, it serves as a trellis upon which new bone can grow.

The pieces of bone that are grafted to the vertebrae in a fusion may come from one or two sources, which surgeons call donor sites. One such site is the iliac crest, the ridge of bone at the top of the pelvis. Some surgeons prefer to use bone from the ilium because it has a rich blood supply, enhancing the chances of a successful fusion. The ilium is also better able to repair itself when bone is taken for a fusion.

The surgeon can get bone from the ilium in the same operation by extending the incision from the spine to the iliac crest on either the right or left side.

The slices of bone used in a spinal fusion may also be taken from the shin bone or tibia. Some surgeons prefer the tibia because it is stronger than the ilium, and patients say it hurts less during recovery, although it always takes a second incision to remove.

The most successful and least painful back fusions use bone that comes from a bone bank. The bone to be used in the fusion may be prepared by one of two methods. It is either removed from a fresh cadaver under sterile conditions, cultured, and preserved by freezing. Or it is removed under unsterile conditions, washed, and then sterilized with ethylene-oxide gas. It is then cultured, and preserved by freezing. Again, the ilium is considered the best bone by surgeons who use a bone bank.

The probability of the implanted bone from a bone bank being properly fused is nearly 100 percent.

The advantages of using a bone bank are obvious. Instead of two operations, the patient only needs one. If the bone bank is not used, grafts are often taken from the patient a day before the spinal fusion is done, or else they are removed during the fusion. The need for two surgeries in two days, or the extended time required for removing bone from the ilium during the fusion can be very hard on a patient who is already experiencing a lot of pain.

Patient recovery time for a fusion that has incorporated bone from a bone bank is dramatically less than one using bone from the patient.

CHEMONUCLEOLYSIS

Chemonucleolysis involves the injection of chemopapain, an enzyme derived from the leaves of the papaya plant, into a herniated disc. The enzyme digests the nucleus pulposus, and eliminates the need for more extensive surgery.

Even though chemonucleolysis has proven to be very effective in over 7,000 cases, the Food and Drug Administration has banned the procedure in the United States. Some states are now passing legislation to restore the procedure.

Diagnosis and treatment are combined during the operation, which is done under general anesthetic. With the patient lying on one side, and using flouroscopic guidance, the surgeon places needles into the nucleus pulposus of the discs that are to be investigated. A radiopaque substance is injected into the suspected discs and a discogram is performed to determine the site of the trouble. When a bad disc is discovered, the radiopaque material is withdrawn. Chemopapain is then injected, drop-by-drop, to digest away the offending portion of the disc. Only the degenerated portion of the nucleus pulposes is dissolved by the enzyme, leaving the annulus fibrosis intact. If the procedure works perfectly, part of the nucleus pulposes will be absorbed by the enzyme and excreted in the patient's urine. The rest will gradually be replaced by fibrous tissue. In effect, chemonucleolysis is supposed to accomplish the same thing as a laminectomy, but without open surgery.

The entire procedure takes about one hour. Band-aids are used for dressing at the points where the needles are inserted. After the first couple of days, the patient is encouraged to walk and engage in hydrotherapy. Hospitalization is required for seven to ten days after the injection, depending on the patient's recovery rate.

Statistics have shown that 65 percent of the patients who have had chemonucleolysis have had good or excellent relief of pain, but two years after injection, the percentage dropped to 42 percent. Compared with laminectomy (with simple disc removal), chemonucleolysis gave about the same short-term and long-range results.

Before you make a decision about surgery, you should evaluate everything involved, including the surgical procedure, hospital facilities, and your surgeon's success rate. You must have confidence in your surgeon and positive feelings about the potential outcome. Doubt and negative attitudes will carry over and extend your recovery period.

You should also develop and carry out a recovery plan that includes diet, exercise, and gradual elimination of medications.

Surgery is a big step, and it involves some risk. But if it is carefully thought out, it can hasten the time when you are no longer restricted by disability and pain.

26. TREATMENT OF
CHRONIC PAIN

If you have experienced back problems, you have undoubtedly experienced pain. The pain may have been prolonged and severe, or moderate and short-lived. The nature and location of your back pain were probably useful in diagnosing the extent of your problems. Even muscle spasm pain protected you against further damage by immobilizing affected parts of your body. But regardless of its beneficial aspects, you—like other bad-back victims—would probably rather be free of pain of any kind.

Acute, short-term pain associated with back strain can be treated with aspirin, massage, rest, and the application of heat. Long-term, debilitating, chronic pain requires much different methods, however.

This chapter discusses the nature and treatment of chronic back pain.

CHRONIC PAIN

Pain experts contend that the average physician hasn't been adequately trained to deal with chronic pain. Too many doctors have failed to recognize that acute, short-term pain and chronic pain are two entirely different phenomena. Because chronic pain has too often been treated like acute pain, narcotic painkillers and other drugs have been used extensively. This has resulted in drug-dependency and other problems for the bad-back sufferers.

Doctors have also been accused of resorting too readily to surgery for the treatment of chronic back pain. Some pain experts, for example, feel there are far too many operations for low-back pain, especially when caused by the pressure of a bulging or degenerated disc, rather than by a disc that has actually ruptured. Some pain experts contend that back pain, and the underlying disc problems, can be treated by other means. The controversy continues, however, with no resolution in sight.

Chronic pain can bring havoc to a person's personality, so the experts try to treat the pain before it starts to control a person's life. One way of dealing with chronic pain is to perform a cordotomy in which nerve fibers that transmit pain are cut. In treating pain in the lower back and legs, for example, surgeons will cauterize the spinothalmic nerve tract above the area where the pain originates. No one really understands why, but the pain-relieving effects of a cordotomy frequently wear off after a year's time, so the operation is usually done only for terminal cancer patients.

Electrical stimulation is one of the newest and fastest growing methods of treating chronic pain. It involves the implantation of fine wire electrodes into the spinal cord above the level of pain. The wires are attached to coin-sized receivers that are implanted beneath the skin of the back. The patient can then use a transmitter to send electrical signals directly into the spine. A control box is used to turn on the stimulator whenever the need to reduce pain arises. In some cases the electrodes are even planted directed into pain areas in the brain.

Several different approaches are used in electrical stimulation, but the principles are generally the same. The pain victim can introduce electrical impulses that have identical or counterbalancing frequency, wave length, or intensity as the nerve impulses that transmit pain. These impulses can either mask or diffuse the pain impulses. Acupuncture is often used as an alternative to electrical stimulation in the treatment of chronic pain, because it shares many of the same principles.

Doctors and researchers will continue their quest for new knowledge about pain; it's causes and treatments. But relief of your chronic pain will depend a great deal on what you can do on your own. Even though you know your pain is there, you can neutralize it if you allow your mind to focus on something else. Your own mental processes could be the most effective chronic-pain treatment you can find.

Too often, people with chronic pain will seek complete inactivity or rest as an escape from pain. Unfortunately, if you take such a passive, inactive approach to your pain, you could end up hurting more, because you won't be able to avoid thinking about your ominous future. If, on the other hand, you remain as active as you possibly can, you will gain added strength and peace of mind just by completing normal day-to-day activities. Being involved in several activities, or completion of even the simplest tasks will have far more positive effects than complete rest. As a matter of fact, activity of any type will have a therapeutic effect on your chronic pain.

PAIN CLINICS

Some of the newer approaches to the treatment of chronic pain are found in the establishment of pain clinics. Anesthesiologists, psychiatrists, neurologists, and other specialists work together in the clinics to find out why their patients hurt and to prescribe treatments that will help eliminate pain. The primary philosophy behind the pain clinics is the recognition that physical, psychological, and social factors are all involved in chronic-pain problems. The treatment of chronic pain has even developed into a new medical specialty called dolorology. It incorporates a wide range of disciplines and treatments, ranging from radical surgery to Transcendental Meditation.

Most pain clinics attempt to decondition pain behavior and teach ways of detracting the mind from thoughts of suffering. One of the first steps taken is to wean the patients from the drugs that have become a major part of their everyday living. This is usually done by prescribing a daily schedule of medication that consists of smaller and smaller amounts of active painkilling ingredients. At the same time, the doctors try to keep the patients from dwelling on pain-related problems.

In the treatment of pain, the clinics rely less on surgery than on other techniques that basically lessen the patients' pain through distraction and substitution. The methods include hypnosis, biofeedback, meditation, and relaxation exercises. If organic conditions are such that surgery is necessary, it will, of course, be recommended.

Many people with bad backs focus entirely on their pain and forget the cause of their problems. Instead of resting, exercising, or doing whatever else is needed to eliminate their pain, they let it take over their lives. This leads them into a series of psychological problems, such as depression, anxiety, and frustration that require a whole new arsenal of treatments.

27. PSYCHOTHERAPY AND RELAXATION

Trying to overcome a bad back can be very stressful. When stress increases, so do tension and anxiety. Together, they can produce painful muscle spasms and harmful emotional states from which it is difficult to escape.

This chapter discusses psychotherapy and relaxation as two ways of overcoming emotional problems that frequently accompany bad backs.

EMOTIONAL RESPONSE TO BACK PROBLEMS

If you have had recurring or prolonged back problems, you have probably experienced frustration, anger, depression, or any of a number of assorted emotions. If your emotional reactions to back problems were severe, frequent, or disabling, you probably wondered what steps you could take to escape from them.

A bruise or common cold will get better because of the body's self-repairing processes. In many cases, satisfactory recoveries take place without professional attention. In the same way, many of the sorrows, anxieties, and nervous disabilities people suffer tend to work themselves out. The grief caused by the death of a loved one and the anxiety caused by the prospect of a major operation are normal and are usually resolved without treatment by a professional. It is, however, very difficult for most people to decide if a given emotional problem is serious enough to require professional treatment.

If your bad-back problems have caused you to experience serious and recurring periods of depression or despair, you are probably at a point of taking some kind of direct action. Your decision to seek or avoid professional help may be distorted, however, by the emotional disorders that are causing you problems. If you rely only on self-diagnosis and treatment, you could bring on even greater problems. You probably need someone to help you make your decision.

There is evidence to indicate that many untreated nervous conditions get better without the services of a professional. Other evidence indicates, however, that untreated nervous conditions get worse and cause greater problems. When professional or psychological treatment is used, about two-thirds of the people show distinct improvement or cure.

Psychotherapy and relaxation are two ways of overcoming some of the emotional problems you may be experiencing with your bad back. The first utilizes the services of a professional, while the second is something you can do on your own.

PSYCHOTHERAPY

Psychotherapy is a general term for describing several different ways of treating emotional and mental ailments. Psychotherapy does not usually involve the use of drugs, operations, shock treatments, or other physical therapies, although these elements may be used in combined forms of treatment. Basically, psychotherapy involves treatment through words and concepts exchanged between a patient and a therapist. The procedure may vary from mental first-aid, in which the patient is reassured and given good advice, to comprehensive modeling of personality and feelings.

People with emotional problems usually seek help in understanding their situation and in getting advice about the next steps to take. The giving of advice and counsel is the most typical form of psychotherapy, and it is often done by parents, teachers, clergymen, lawyers, physicians, and psychotherapists. Most psychotherapy consists of face-to-face discussions between a patient and a therapist who may have been trained as a psychiatrist, psychologist, or social worker.

There are two major threats to mental health, both of which are encountered by people with bad backs. The first is excessive conflict, characterized by feelings of stress, tension, and anxiety. The second is isolation from other people, with feelings of loneliness and rejection.

The psychotherapist seeks, on one hand, to help the patient break the deadlock of emotional conflicts, and on the other hand to help in achieving more satisfactory interpersonal relationships.

The choice of treatment or no treatment, at least in the case of minor emotional ailments, is more or less up to the patient, although professional advice may be needed to make a sound decision. The family doctor is a primary resource even though only a few family doctors are capable of making detailed psychological diagnoses. More often than not, physicians will prescribe tranquilizing drugs rather than delve into the psychological roots of a problem. Patients with obvious emotional problems will generally be referred to competent practitioners who are more qualified to treat psychological rather than physical disorders.

There is a degree of risk involved with psychotherapy. An incorrect diagnosis of an emotional disorder can be as dangerous to both the patient and the practitioner as an incorrect diagnosis of a bad-back condition. Therefore, it is very important for the therapist to completely understand the patient's situation. If physical disorders are the basic cause, they need to be carefully and completely explained.

RELAXATION

If you elect to work out your emotional and mental ailments by yourself, you may want to examine techniques that help you relax.

Meditation is probably the most popular of many different approaches. Meditation and other deep-relaxation techniques became more widely accepted by the medical community after Dr. Herbert Benson of Harvard University measured the physiological changes that occurred within the human body during relaxation. He noted a significant decrease in the rate of metabolism and a reduction of lactate in the blood. The reactions to meditation and relaxation that Dr. Benson found were exactly opposite to those produced by the body when it is subjected to stress and anxiety. Dr. Benson called the physiological changes the "relaxation response".

The Relaxation Response. The four basic conditions required to elicit the relaxation response are described here.

1. *A Quiet Environment:* You should choose a quiet, calm, and tranquil environment with few distractions. A quiet room is suitable, as is a place of worship.

2. *A Mental Device:* To shift the mind from logical, externally-oriented thought, a constant stimulus, such as a sound, word, or phrase should be repeated silently or aloud. Fixed gazing at an object can also serve this purpose. Since one of the major difficulties in eliciting the relaxation response is mind wandering, the repetition of the sound, word, or phrase helps break the train of distracting thoughts.

3. *A Passive Attitude:* When distracting thoughts occur, they should be disregarded, and attention should be redirected to the mental device. You should not worry about how well you are performing the technique, because this may prevent relaxation from occuring. A passive attitude is perhaps the most important element in eliciting the relaxation response. Distracting thoughts will occur but you should not worry about them. Simply put them aside and return to the repetition of the mental device. Like an unwelcome intruder, distractions will return again and again as you try to relax.

4. *A Comfortable Position:* You should be comfortable to avoid undue muscular tension. Many people sit in a comfortable chair, and some use the cross-legged position of Yoga. With your bad back, you may find lying down to be the most comfortable position, but you must stay awake and not let yourself fall asleep.

HOW TO RELAX

Each time you seek to bring about the relaxation response, you should follow a standard procedure, such as the one suggested here.

1. Sit or lie in a comfortable position.
2. Close your eyes, unless you are using a visual object for your mental device.

3. Deeply relax all your muscles, beginning at your feet and progressing up to your face.
4. Breathe easily and naturally through your nose. As you breathe out, silently say the word or phrase that you have chosen. It should be easily repeated and sound natural to you.
5. Continue the relaxation response for 10 or 20 minutes. Don't set an alarm since that may startle you and cause you to lose the relaxed effect you have gained. Sit quietly for a few minutes before you get up so you can enjoy the tranquility.
6. Don't worry about your success in achieving a deep level of relaxation. If you maintain a passive attitude, relaxation will occur at its own pace. With practice, the relaxation response should come about with little effort if done once or twice a day. Don't attempt to elicit the response within two hours after a meal since the digestive processes may interfere with your ability to reach deep levels of relaxation.

Another relaxation technique you may wish to use is prayer from your religious tradition. Choose a prayer that incorporates the four elements necessary to bring forth the relaxation response. Prayers are one way to remedy an inner incompleteness and to reduce inner discord.

Stress and tension can have a devastating effect on your recovery program. By dealing directly with the forces in your environment that create stress and tension, you will be able to take significant steps toward overcoming your bad back.

28. OTHER TREATMENTS

There are almost as many ways of treating a bad back as there are causes of back problems. The more traditional methods of treatment have been covered in previous chapters. This chapter describes the use of manipulation, traction, corsets and braces, biofeedback training, and zone therapy as additional treatments for back problems.

Manipulation, traction, and corsets and braces are included because of their extensive use in the treatment of bad backs. Biofeedback is discussed because it is a new and promising treatment. Zone therapy is mentioned to illustrate the different kinds of treatment that exist.

MANIPULATION

Manipulation involves the movement of bones and supporting structures to correct dislocations and subluxations. Dislocation is the separation of bones in a joint from their normal position, and a subluxation is a partial separation. They are generally caused by an acute injury.

The joints in the body are held together by ligaments, cartilage, and other tissues. Movable joints, like those involving vertebrae, are encased in joint capsules that are covered with ligaments and filled with fluids that facilitate movement.

If your back pain has come on suddenly and improved with rest, you may possibly have suffered a dislocation or subluxation. It may have happened when you moved suddenly or lifted a heavy object and placed an excessive strain on your intervertebral joints. If, on the other hand, your pain has come on over an extended period of time and seems to get worse whether you rest or not, your problem may involve other structures.

Manipulation stretches the surrounding tissue enough to unlock the joint and allow the displaced bones to return to their normal position. If manipulation is successful, the victim will often experience an immediate and dramatic relief from pain, because muscle spasms that often are involved will stop. But the stretched ligaments will not spring back like an elastic or rubber band. They contract slowly over time, during which the patient should rest and remain quiet. If not allowed to retract normally, the ligaments may stretch again, and a cycle of subluxation, manipulation, and stretching will recur until the ligaments can no longer hold the joint together.

Manipulation is done by chiropractors, osteopaths, and an increasing number of medical doctors. In a typical chiropractic adjustment or surgical reduction of a vertebral joint, the patient will be positioned face up on a table. The patient's right shoulder will be held down by the manipulator's left hand. The right side of the patient's pelvis will then be rotated as far as possible to the left, taking up the slack in the affected joint. The manipulator will then press downward and to the left on the patient's hip. A sudden downward thrust will separate the dislocated joint surfaces and allow them to return to their normal positions.

Sometimes a crack or pop is heard during manipulation. This means a vertebral joint has moved or a joint capsule has stretched. The same thing occurs when you crack your knuckles. It does not mean that a slipped disc has popped back in place.

If you have a herniated disc that is protruding out into the spinal canal, manipulation may be the worst treatment you could possibly have. Movement of vertebrae that are in proper position may pinch nerves that are already abused, and additional damage may result to either a nerve or a disc.

Like other treatments, manipulation should only be utilized after a thorough diagnosis has been completed by a medical doctor who is trained to detect all sorts of disorders that may be causing intense back pain. Manipulation without proper diagnosis can have very serious consequences. This is especially true if a herniated disc or diseased organ is causing the pain.

TRACTION

Traction is another form of deliberate manipulation. If it is applied over a sufficient period of time, it can produce the same benefits as manipulation. And it is generally safer than manipulation because of the absence of sudden and dramatic movements in painful regions of the back.

Traction is not intended to stretch or pull your vertebrae apart to allow a herniated disc to slip back into place as many people believe. Normal pelvic traction, using 10 to 15 pound weights, may do little more than serve as a restraint for keeping you in bed. It will raise your pelvis and reduce the curve in your spine, thereby relieving pressure on a herniated disc and curtailing muscle spasms. But strategically placed pillows can have almost the same effect on spinal curves, and they are far more comfortable than traction.

Pelvic traction as illustated in figure 22, utilizes a girdlelike belt that wraps around your waist and hips. Straps are attached to the sides and to a nylon cord that hangs over the end of your bed. Various sized weights are attached to the end of the nylon cord, and the traction is maintained for several hours at a time. The maximum weight that can be used in pelvic traction is about 15 pounds. Anything over that will pull you right off the end of your bed.

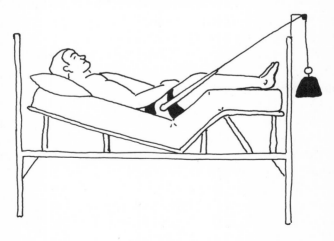

FIGURE 22. PELVIC TRACTION

Special equipment has been designed to handle weights up to 200 pounds. It involves a series of straps that are wrapped around your chest and attached to a fixed object about your head. Another set of straps, to which weights are attached, is wrapped around your hips. In theory, when muscles are pulled on long enough, they fatigue, allowing joint structures to stretch. As traction is relieved, the subluxated joint will come back together into its proper position.

CORSETS AND BRACES

The practice of making and fitting corsets, braces, and appliances for treating disorders of joints and muscles is called orthotics. The specifications for such devices follow prescriptions written by qualified medical practitioners. There are probably hundreds of different wearable devices that a person may use in the treatment of a bad back.

Braces used to support the lumbar spine are based on a three-point pressure principle, with the supporting pressures coming from three directions. One example might involve a backward thrust against the front of the hipbones or pelvis, a second backward thrust against the rib cage and the front of the chest, and a forward thrust against the lower back and lumbar spine.

The specific location and direction of the three pressure points may vary. In the Williams lordosis brace, for example, there are two forward pressure points at the back—the lower thoracic spine and the sacral region—opposing a single backward force at the lower abdomen. In each case, however, the sum of the two points in one direction should equal the opposing single force, which should be placed approximately midway between the other two.

There are instances where using a corset or brace is essential, such as after a severe injury to the spine. In cases where muscles have become paralyzed, a brace to support the back may be unavoidable. Patients with scoliosis often need a special brace to help correct curvature of the spine. Some patients may have to wear a corset permanently if they are unable to strengthen stomach muscles through exercise because of a severe heart condition, hernia, or other problem.

Back braces and other supportive devices should not be used

indiscriminately, because over time they tend to weaken the muscles that support the spine. They should be considered a temporary aid, to be worn only until stomach and back muscles are strengthened. As long as corsets and braces are used to support the abdominal muscles, the muscles will not be used. They will tend to atrophy and weaken, increasing the likelihood of more back pain.

If you ever hope to overcome your bad back, it is imperative that you maintain strong back and abdominal muscles and not let them fall prey to the inactivity that results from the use of braces. Too many people unnecessarily depend on braces and other supportive devices, and the longer they wear them, the longer they will need them.

BIOFEEDBACK

Biofeedback teaches individuals to control bodily processes by exercising the powers of the mind. Variations in the bodily processes are not ordinarily perceived by the conscious mind. Now, however, biofeedback techniques can display previously unavailable information through visual or auditory means. This information is used by individuals to control or change bodily processes that were previously thought to be ungovernable by conscious thought.

Biofeedback has already proved useful in helping individuals relax in the face of stress. One successful application involves the treatment of patients with chronic pain that is induced by stress and muscle tension. The patients are connected to a machine that monitors muscle tension and "feeds back" the level of existing tension by emitting a series of electronic beeps. When the patient's muscles become tense, the sounds increase in volume and frequency. They decrease in volume and frequency when the muscles relax. With practice, patients can relax tense muscles by responding to and slowing down the electronic beeps. As the patients consciously slow down the auditory signals, muscle tension is also reduced. Eventually, patients learn to induce deep muscle relaxation without relying on machine feedback.

Most doctors and laypeople agree that emotional upset makes pain worse. If patients can remain relaxed in the face of such upsets, their pain may actually be reduced. By focusing on the physical pain—

through biofeedback techniques—rather than the psychological discomfort of a stressful situation, patients might also lessen their pain awareness.

ZONE THERAPY

Zone therapy is based on the notion that pressure on certain parts of the body can relieve discomfort from disease conditions that are far removed from the point where the pressure is applied. Zone therapists suggest, for example, that pressure applied to points on the fingers, hands, or feet can relieve internal disease, discomfort, and pain at distant sites, such as the head. In this regard, zone therapy is similar to acupuncture, in which the insertion of needles into certain areas of the body may relieve pain at distant sites.

29. SUMMARY OF PART III

It is essential for you to know what is wrong with your back and what you can do to correct it. Diagnosis is the key to effective treatment, because no cure can accurately be prescribed for any condition until the cause is clearly understood. Treatment of back problems can vary greatly among the specialists who deal with bad backs. Two practitioners within the same specialty can use different procedures for performing the same diagnosis and treatment. If you get lost trying to understand what others are doing to you, you will lose control of your destiny, and you will find it very difficult to overcome your bad back.

Part III describes a variety of procedures for diagnosing back problems, from physical examinations and the assessment of pain, to the use of sophisticated chemical and electronic analysis. It describes some of the benefits that exercise can provide, as well as some of the dangers that should be avoided. It also suggests several specific exercises that can be very helpful in overcoming back problems.

Part III also discusses the nature of back surgery and describes three of the most common surgical techniques that are used to correct back problems. It also discusses the nature and treatment of chronic pain. It discusses psychotherapy and relaxation as two ways of overcoming emotional problems that frequently accompany bad backs. Finally, Part III describes the use of manipulation, traction, corsets and braces, biofeedback training, and zone therapy as additional treatments for back problems.

BIBLIOGRAPHY

Benson, Herbert (with Miriam Klipper). *The Relaxation Response.* New York: William Morrow and Company, Inc., 1975.

Berland, Theodore and Addison, Robert. *Living With Your Bad Back.* New York: St. Martin's Press, Inc., 1972

Brody, Jane E. "Experts: A Few Simple Tips Stop Most Backaches." *Minneapolis Tribune*, 19 May 1977.

"Chemonucleolysis:Better Than Laminectomy?". *Journal of the American Medical Association.* 16 April 1973, pp. 287-96

Clark, Matt. "The New War On Pain." *Newsweek,* 25 April 1977, pp. 48-58

Clements, H. *What To Do About A Bad Back and Disc Trouble.* New York: Drake Publishers, 1972

Cloward, Ralph B. "Lesions of the Intervertebral Discs and Their Treatment by Interbody Fusion Methods." *Clinical Orthopaedics*, No. 27, 1963, pp. 51-77

————. "Multiple Ruptured Discs." *Annals of Surgery,* August 1955

————. *Ruptured Lumbar Intervertebral Discs.* Randolph, MA: Codman & Shurtless, Inc., n.d.

————. "Vertebral Body Fusion for Ruptured Lumbar Discs: A Roentgenographic Study." *American Journal of Surgery,* December 1955, pp. 969-976

Cooley, Donald., ed. *Better Homes and Gardens Family Medical Guide.* New York: Meredith Press, 1964.

Digby, John W. "Management of Low Back Pain." *Modern Medicine,* 23 October 1967, pp. 49-58

Everroad, James M. *How To Flatten Your Stomach.* Los Angeles: Price/Stern/Sloan, 1978

157

Fahrni,W. Harry. *Backache Relieved Through New Concepts of Posture.* Springfield, IL: C. C. Thomas, 1966

Finneson, Bernard and Freese, Arthur S. *Dr. Finneson On Low Back Pain.* New York: G. P. Putnam's Sons, 1975

Friedman, Lawrence and Galton, Lawrence. *Freedom From Backaches.* New York: Simon and Schuster, 1973

Friedman, Meyer and Rosenman, Ray H. *Type A Behavior and Your Heart.* New York: Fawcette Crest Books, 1974

Hearn, Editha. *You Are As Young As Your Spine.* Garden City, NY: Doubleday & Co., 1967

Homola, Samuel. *Backache: Home Treatment and Prevention.* West Wyack, NY: Parker Publishing Company, 1968

Inglis, Brian. *The Book of the Back.* New York: Herst Books, 1978.

Ishmael, William K. and Shorbe, Howard B. *Care of the Back.* 2nd ed. Philadelphia: J. R. Lippincott Company, 1969

————.*Care of the Back, Industrial Edition.* Philadelphia: J. R. Lippincott Company, 1969

Klein, Frederick C. "My Aching Back." *Wall Street Journal.* 26 May 1972, p. 1

Kopell, Harvey P. and Kester, Nancy C. *Help for Your Aching Back!* New York: Grosset & Dunlap, 1969

Krames, Lawrence A. *The Back Owner's Manual.* Los Angeles: Price/Stern/Sloan, 1977

Kraus, Hans. *Backache, Stress, and Tension: Their Cause, Prevention, and Treatment.* New York: Simon and Schuster, 1965

Leach, Robert E. "Disc Disease, Spondyolysis, and Spondylolithesis." *Athletic Training.* Spring 1977, pp. 13-17

Neimark, Paul G. *A Doctor Discusses Care of the Back.* Chicago: Budlong Press Company, 1975

Nolen, William A. "What to do About Pain that Won't Go Away." *McCalls,* October 1978, pp. 82-84, 216

Nordby, Eugene J. "Chymopapain for the Treatment of Back Pain and Sciatica". Mimeographed. Madison, WI: University of Wisconsin, n.d.

Root, Leon and Kiernan, Thomas. *Oh, My Aching Back.* New York: David McKay Company, Inc., 1973

Rothenberg, Robert E. *The New Understanding Surgery: The Complete Surgical Guide.* New York: New American Library, 1974

Scarf, Maggie. "Husbands in Crisis." *McCalls,* June 1972, pp. 76-77

Sheehy, Gail. *Passages: Predictable Crises of Adult Life.* New York: E. P. Dutton & Company, 1974

Shuman, David and Staab, George R. *Your Aching Back and What You Can Do About It.* New York: Gramercy, 1968

Stern, Jess. *Dr. Thompson's New Way For You To Cure Your Aching Back.* Garden City, NY: Doubleday & Co., Inc., 1973

Thompson, H. J. *Overcoming Back Trouble.* New York: Prentice Hall, 1953

Wayne, Jerry. *The Bad Back Book.* New York: Prentice Hall, 1953

Williams, Gurney. "Your Aching Back." *Family Health/ Today's Health,* March 1977

Zauner, Renate. *Speaking of: Backaches.* New York: Consolidated Book Publishers, 1978

INDEX

161

hip hyperextension exercise: 132
history, medical: 57, 116
hostility: 107-108
  as factor of depression: 107-108
  toward others: 109
  toward sexual partner: 67
husband-wife relationships: 47

iliac crest: 137
illustrations, importance of: 85
immobilization: 30, 31
infections and tumors: 2, 16, 120
  and surgery: 133
  see also arthritis
information *see* knowledge
injury *see* trauma
internal medicine: 83
  and diagnosis: 83
  and surgery: 83
internist: 83, 116
intervertebral disc *see* disc

joint capsule: 149, 150

kinesiologists: 26
knee to chest raise exercise: 128
knowledge (information)
  about drugs and alcohol:
    192-195
  about sexual problems: 69-70
  about your condition:
  from others: 59-60
  need for: 3, 7-8, 85
  self-help books: 57-58, 109
  sharing: 59, 86

lactic acid and muscle spasms: 29,
  31
lamina(e): 134, 135
laminectomy
  combination with fusion: 135
  compared to chemonucleolysis:
    138
  effect of: 135

procedure for: 134-135
  success rate for: 135
lateral trunk stretch exercise: 127
leg pains: 19
  see also sciatica
lifting: 97
  and bending: 21
  importance of muscles in: 26
  problems in: 97
  proper way: 101-103
  research on: 97
ligaments: 10, 32-34
  annulus fibrosus: 17, 19, 21, 23
  anterior and posterior
    longitudinal: 33
  damage to: 27, 33-34
  facet capsule: 33
  importance of: 7
  in manipulation: 150
  in surgery: 135, 136
  interspinous: 32
  intertransverse: 32
  ligamentum flavum: 33
liniments and ointments: 31
lordosis *see* swayback
lumbago: 1, 39
lumbar vertebrae: 9-10

manipulation: 149-150
  accidental: 30
  and muscle spasms: 30
  chiropractic: 82-83
  dangers in: 150
  deliberate: 30, 150, 151
  osteopathy and: 84
marital stress: 71-75
  and midlife problems: 47
  and social life: 77
massage: 41, 69
masturbation: 69
mattresses: 99, 106
medication(s)
  and exercise: 124, 125
  and muscle spasms: 30, 31